Praise from others in the field for *The Educated Heart*:

A candid, informative presentation on the major ethical issues that bodyworkers face every day... Openly discusses topics that are commonly confronted but rarely talked about. An invaluable resource for both new and veteran bodyworkers. — **Dianne Polseno, LPN, LMT: Ethics columnist,** *Massage Therapy Journal*; **Clinical Massage department head, Bancroft School; Former chairperson, AMTA Ethics**

This book speaks directly to issues of practice and professionalism that massage students and massage therapists are concerned and often confused about. Nina McIntosh makes a challenging subject accessible, even inviting, by using many real life examples and by bringing her substantial compassion and humor to questions of how and why we make mistakes, and how, in the end, establishing clear boundaries allows us to do more effective work with our clients. — **Lucy Liben, M.S., LMT: Dean for Academic Affairs, Swedish Institute, New York, New York**

The Educated Heart provides a clear and engaging treatment of the complex psychological and ethical issues between bodyworkers and their clients. It should be required reading for students and professionals. — **Alan Fogel, Ph.D.: Professor of Psychology, University of Utah; Rosen Method bodywork student; Salt Lake City, Utah**

Nina McIntosh speaks with a voice that has an assurance and a respect that makes me want to listen. Reading *The Educated Heart* is like going back to school and filling in the gaps in one's education about professional boundaries and ethics. I highly recommend this book as a tool for self-exploration and fine-tuning our ethical practices and how better to serve the needs of our clients. — **Robert Litman: International Continuum Teacher; Head of the Movement Department and Movement Integration Teacher for the Desert Institute of the Healing Arts, Tucson, Arizona; Certified Advanced Duggan/French Approach Movement Teacher**

I would recommend this book to my students. The author has incredible insight into human character. Her psychological background shows clearly and richly throughout the book. — **Kristina Shaw: Director, Healing Hands School of Massage; Philadelphia, Pennsylvania**

Intelligent, to-the-point and very clear... Nina guides us to understand what goes on under the surface in our practices. She suggests ways to establish boundaries, the do's and don'ts of caregiving, when to say "yes," when to say "no" and how to practice self-care. With sensitivity she helps us understand the dynamics of the client/practitioner connection, the pitfalls inherent in dual relationships and how our clients project onto us—often without their or our awareness. A valuable and much needed contribution to the somatic field. — **Rob Bauer, CSW: Master Rubenfeld Synergist; Imago Relationship Therapist; Senior Faculty Member and Supervisor of the Rubenfeld Synergy® Method; Salem, New York**

I believe that relationship is the essence of healing. In *The Educated Heart*, Nina provides the massage therapy student or practicing therapist with a book that speaks beyond technique to what is truly the "heart of the matter," the therapeutic relationship. — **Carol P. Burke, M.S., CRNP: Former Director of Education, Baltimore School of Massage, Baltimore, Maryland; Instructor, University of Maryland School of Medicine, Complementary Medicine Program**

In an easy style, with great clarity, Nina McIntosh enlightens us to the complex labyrinth of issues lurking under the banner of ethics, professionalism and boundaries.... A practical book with sound information, thoroughly grounded in knowledge and experience, drawn from the wisdom of many seasoned practitioners. I will certainly include this book as required reading on my training course and recommend it to long-standing practitioners to refresh their energy on this cornerstone of a responsible and successful practice. — **Vivien Schapera: Director of Alexander Technique of Cincinnati; Cincinnati, Ohio**

The Educated Heart reflects Nina McIntosh's painstaking effort to fairly discuss the ethical dilemmas and minefields associated with today's bodywork. I agree with her message that clients give us their vulnerability and trust and deserve our respect and compassion. This helpful book spells out the ways practitioners can show their clients that respect and compassion. — **Charles Wiltsie, LMT: Ethics instructor for men; Higganum, Connecticut**

THE EDUCATED HEART

Professional Guidelines for Massage Therapists,
Bodyworkers and Movement Teachers

BY NINA McINTOSH

Cartoon Illustrations by Mari Gayatri Stein

Decatur Bainbridge Press

The Educated Heart

Published in the United States of America by Decatur Bainbridge Press, Memphis, Tennessee. For information, contact DBainbrdge@aol.com, (877) 327-0600

First Printing, 1999
Second Printing, 2000
ISBN 0-9674122-0-X
Library of Congress Catalogue Card Number: 99-93428

Cover art: "Aslipah, Disguised As A River, Was Lowered Close To The Water By His Friends." Artist: Dolph Smith.

Handmade paper, original piece 18" x 24," Date: 1987. From the collection of and with the kind permission of Kathy Albers, Albers Gallery, Memphis, Tennessee.

This piece is part of the saga of the heroic journey of Aslipah, a paper airplane, and his struggle to prevail. Aslipah challenges the stereotype of being just "a slip of paper" and is embarked on a quest for the elusive meaning of life. Just as Aslipah is a symbol for everywoman/man's personal drama, his story is an apt metaphor for the journey of the manual therapies to reach a position of recognition and enlightenment.

Cover design: Amy Sharp
Text design: Kelli Glazier

*Dedicated to the memory of my parents
who were always waiting
for me to get a real job.*

Table of Contents

✖

Usage

For any writer conscious of gender sensitivities who wants to produce easily-read sentences, the dilemma of the third person singular is daunting. The question is whether to use "she" or "he" to mean all people and thus to exclude the other sex or whether to use the awkward "he/she" or "she/he." In *The Educated Heart*, the dilemma has been resolved by alternating between the two gender pronouns and between the two variations of "he/she and "she/he." No malice is intended when either "he" or "she" is associated with an unethical practitioner or an annoying client—it's just the luck of the draw.

Remaining sensitive to the various modalities within the manual therapies and finding a universal name for what we do is equally daunting. (Feldenkrais and Alexander practitioners, for instance, prefer to be called teachers, and rightfully object to being categorized under bodyworkers.) Although it may not thoroughly suit everyone, I have settled on the term "manual therapist" as an umbrella term to include massage therapists, bodyworkers, movement educators, practitioners of the Oriental methods and practitioners who work with energy fields. For the sake of readability, I have occasionally used "bodywork" or "bodyworker" as a generic term. When I use the terms, "our work" or "our profession," I mean all of the manual therapies.

Foreword

For years, decades even, there have been no overview books covering the complexities of professional boundaries for those who are healers and helpers who communicate with the blessed body.

But now, with this new work by Nina McIntosh, brand-new massage students and advanced bodyworkers, massage therapists, and movement teachers alike, including practitioners of such disciplines as Feldenkrais, Alexander technique, Rosen Method bodywork, and others, will be likely to find this book not only useful and comprehensive, but also recognize and feel "companioned" by the "inside skivvie" stories of the trade—told as only one from the inner circle of the profession can.

Too often, the newly graduated, the inexperienced, and/or the temporarily stressed practitioner is left to find their own way, to make guesses about what is important or appropriate, rather than having available a reference they can consult for reliable guidelines. This work puts so much of that to rest by giving the practitioner reassuring vignettes, examples, and plentiful advice about what to do, and more importantly, what <u>not</u> to do. Here the author reveals critical information about cherishing the therapeutic relationship, that is, taking care of the details, boundaries and nourishments of running a practice and serving one's clients. She generously shares solutions to many real-life conundrums, impasses and other sensitive situations that face every professional.

Also, extending the natural wit and wisdom of the book are the illustrations. In the tradition of James Thurber and Nicole Hollander and other psychological cartoonists, the witty and charming cartoons of Mari Gayatri Stein grace this book. You will likely recognize yourself and others you know in these artful little gems.

When I first heard this book was in the works, I felt gladdened to know that the sharing of such important information would be available to all the deeply committed bodyworkers of the world, and equally heartened to know that an insightful and sensitive woman would be writing it. Nina McIntosh has over twenty-six years of experience as either a bodyworker or a psychiatric social worker. She writes for the caring bodyworker who strives to protect both psyche and <u>soma</u>, that is, the body and soul of the individual who trustingly comes to the practitioner for help, strengthening, and a calming environs. This long-needed work is as much a companion for the journey as it is a book. And like a good companion, it is not only fascinating and lively— it is also that most important of all qualities— it is <u>useful</u>.

Clarissa Pinkola Estés, Ph.D.
Diplomate Jungian Analyst
Grievance Board Chair, State of Colorado

Introduction

✖

When I first started out as a bodyworker in 1978, I wasn't concerned about acting like a "professional." In fact, I thought it might be a good thing to avoid.

I had just fled a job as a psychiatric social worker in a stuffy private mental hospital where "professional" often meant acting detached and distant. I was drawn by the seeming simplicity and earthiness of massage therapy.

At that time massage therapy was in its early stages of development as a legitimate career choice. It was struggling for dignity and credibility in the field of health care, as it still is in some parts of the country. Perhaps because of this, some massage schools appeared to have modeled themselves on medical schools: they focused mainly on teaching anatomy and technique, with little mentioned about creating a safe environment for clients or about appropriate relationships. If anything was said, it was as a casual aside. That was the state of the art in the late '70s.

Although my previous training had made me familiar with standards of practice for clinical social workers, I didn't think the same standards would apply to massage therapy. After all, we weren't delving into peoples' psyches, were we? I thought people were simply coming to us to relax tight muscles.

Massage therapists who I knew then were often casual about the way they ran their practices. None of us imagined we had to put thought into issues such as having friends for clients or working out of our homes. We were in the vanguard of a new approach to health and healing—"holistic" was a new word and a fresh concept. Just as I wanted to distance myself from the chilly and unnatural professional behavior of the psychiatric setting, others entering the alternative health fields sought to distance themselves from an increasingly cold and technical medical world.

And so, like many others at the time, I embarked on my bodywork career thinking of myself as a free spirit. I was going to throw aside the shackles of my uptight training and be warm, human and healing. People would come to me tied in knots and leave refreshed and renewed. It would be an uncomplicated way to make a living and to help people at the same time—or so it seemed.

It wasn't that simple. Some clients did come in knots and leave in clouds of bliss. Others never seemed to relax or let go. And while some clients became regulars, others would come once and then disappear. It was harder than I had expected to keep a practice afloat.

I didn't know what was wrong or how to fix it, but parts of my practice weren't working. Sometimes I blamed the clients: they were too "conventional" to understand the benefits of massage. Sometimes I blamed myself: maybe I wasn't "caring" enough—whatever that meant. Most of the time it was just a mystery to me.

Hoping for Magic

After three years of a moderately successful massage practice, I decided to get more training. Going through the basic

Rolfing series as a client had been a process of major transformation and self-discovery for me. Re-aligning tissue seemed like magic, and I had the secret hope that this additional training would also magically clear up the problems I was having with clients.

Well, not exactly. At that time, the Rolf Institute, like every other school in the alternative health field, didn't give much weight to teaching professional standards and basic boundary guidelines. The anti-establishment influence of the '60s still lingered—ironically so. Although we thought of ourselves as mavericks, manual therapy schools mimicked the medical schools by teaching as though the fine points of relationship and professional setting didn't matter. What students did learn of professionalism, we learned by example—and I was lucky my teachers provided good role models. (Since then, as with many schools, things have changed at the Rolf Institute and more is taught about professional boundaries and client dynamics.)

Solving a Mystery

In 1982, two years into my practice as a Rolfer, I went to a seminar that started me down the path to writing this book. The lecturer was Nan Narboe, a psychotherapist from Portland, Oregon, and her message was an eye-opener for me: we could be the best aligners of connective tissue in the world, but clients will judge our competence more by the way *our practices* are aligned. They gauge whether they can feel safe with us by how professional we are and how we deal with boundaries. They may react to feeling unsafe by getting ornery, closing up, or never coming back.

She explained the psychodynamics of the situation and why errors in the framework* make clients uncomfortable, although they may not be conscious of the reason. Even if the type of bodywork is not psychologically oriented, being touched can bring up old unresolved feelings. The body contains the unconscious, and memories that we've ignored or hidden from ourselves. Also, because of the perceived power difference between us and our clients, it is important our clients be able to trust us, if they are to relax. It's up to us—through the way we structure our practices and how we handle our relationships with clients—to help them feel secure enough to be receptive to our work.

Sitting in the audience, I wondered if this was the answer to the "disappearing client" mystery. I remembered clients who had abruptly stopped coming and clients I had never been able to reach. With each one, I could remember something I'd done that may have made them uneasy— giving unsolicited advice, not being clear about money or perhaps not being attentive enough to a special problem. In my casual approach to professionalism, what I thought was naturalness was often self-indulgence. Like most bodyworkers, I hadn't made colossal errors of judgment that sent clients screaming from my office, but I looked back at my lack of sensitivity and winced.

It began to dawn on me that being professional didn't mean hiding behind a facade of superiority. Instead, it meant being consistent and conscientious. Boundaries didn't create walls between client and practitioner—they helped clients feel safe.

---

*Definition on page 228.

After that seminar, I vowed to be more conscious of boundaries and framework. I noticed that when I was attentive to them, my practice hummed along with few disturbances. When I was careless, it was reflected in clients who just happened to forget their appointments, clients who complained, clients who couldn't seem to relax, or those who simply never returned.

The Other Side of the Table

After I had been practicing for several years, my life took a turn that made my musings about the benefits of professionalism far more personal. I became a needy client myself—in pain, sick or both. This lasted for the next ten years. During that decade, as I dealt with one health issue after another, I learned more about the importance of boundaries and framework in the therapeutic relationship*, not from being a practitioner (although I kept a small practice), but from being the client on the table.

My first in a series of health challenges was a TMJ problem, an imbalance in the temporo-mandibular joint that impinges on nerves and sometimes causes, as it did for me, a constant dreadful pain. It was awful and I was desperate to make the pain go away. In the process of trying to make it go away, I became the bodyworker's worst nightmare—a hypersensitive client in pain who wants to be "fixed."

One of my lessons during that time was that I could be a client-from-hell one day and an easy-going client the next, depending on how I was treated. What made the difference was what happened *before* I was ever on the table. When a

*Definition on page 229.

client feels as frightened and frantic as I did, small boundary or framework errors seem like major signs of incompetence or indifference. Soothing, non-judgmental words in peaceful offices were vacations in the mountains. Careless words and sloppy boundaries were elephant feet, trampling my nervous system. I became painfully aware of the ways otherwise skilled practitioners create "difficult" clients.

Mysterious and Undocumented

Stressed from years of physical pain, I came down with what I thought was the flu. When I still had it six months later, I realized that something else was going on. Eventually I was diagnosed with what is currently called Chronic Fatigue Syndrome—an illness that causes, among other things, constant flu-like aches and pains, low grade fevers, and debilitating exhaustion. It became a struggle just to get to the grocery store.

One of the major boundary mistakes a person with an illness runs into, particularly a mysterious and undocumented illness, is presumed expertise. Practitioners who knew little about the illness or about me thought that they could tell me just what I had done wrong to get sick and just what would make me well.

The practitioners who were the most helpful were the ones who listened—simply listened without judgment and without offering advice. They showed compassionate curiosity and were conscientious and attentive. They started sessions on time, stuck to their area of expertise and said things like, "I'm sorry you're sick. What is it like for you?"

Renewed Conviction

My concerns about feeling safe became even more sharply focused when my family suffered a sudden and dramatic tragedy in the fall of 1988. My elderly parents, whose placid and comfortable lives had provided a stable anchor for me over the years, were brutally assaulted in their home and left for dead. They survived with head injuries that turned them into children who needed constant care. Profoundly shaken, I returned to my home town to live with them and supervise their care. What I thought might be a few months lasted seven years.

The shock of the sudden violence and the constant and stressful demands of being a caregiver took another kind of toll on me. Full-blown adult shell shock renders a person very sensitive to the environment. It reverberates to earlier insecurities, which intensifies the need to feel safe.

During those painful years, I appreciated those practitioners who realized that I was, well, a little nuts—and that whatever was going on with me, it wasn't about them. For instance, they understood that my need to fuss with the details, to get the music turned down or the music turned up or the room warmer or the room cooler, wasn't a lack of confidence in them. My world had been turned upside down and there had to be some place where I could feel safe and, at least in small ways, in charge of my environment.

Healing and Boundaries

After my parents died, I realized that I had shut down in order to deal with a terrible situation. I had become a gray and lifeless ghost. I knew I needed a safe environment to coax me out—somewhere I could feel free enough to concentrate on my own issues and safe enough to deal with the deeply-held trauma of those painful years.

I had been in the Rolfing community a long time and knew many of my colleagues well. I had socialized with them; I had disagreed with them; I had heard gossip about them. My boundaries with other Rolfers were pretty much shot full of holes. It had nothing to do with skill; there just wasn't any way that I could go to a colleague without feeling self-conscious. It had all become too entangled. This happens with anyone who has been part of a particular bodywork community for a long time, and like many other bodyworkers, I solved the problem by crossing over to another brand of work—Rosen Method bodywork, a gentle method of working with restrictions in breathing.

When I began to go to week-long Rosen Method Intensives, I found that the boundaries were crystal clear: I had no previous relationship with any of the staff or other students and they only knew about me what I chose to tell them. I didn't have to impress anyone or keep up an image. There was no agenda other than my own personal work. As a result, the experience was as transformational as my first ten sessions of Rolfing. It reinforced the desire in me to write this book.

Educating the Heart

My positive experiences were with Rolfing and Rosen Method bodywork, but any brand of the manual therapies* can be more effective when the setting is safe, when care is

---

*Definition on page 228.

taken with framework, when dual relationships* are avoided and clients are free to focus on themselves.

In the past two decades, the somatic practices have become increasingly aware of the importance of professionalism—maintaining good boundaries, ethics and framework. During that time, my awareness about the need for professionalism came from my years as a practitioner, my painful years as a wounded client and finally, my years of healing as a client-on-the-mend. My experiences brought home to me in a very personal way that the subject of professionalism isn't a dry, theoretical one. Safe spaces and good boundaries can touch clients' hearts and ease their spirits.

*Definition on page 228.

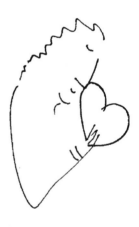

The Educated Heart

Chapter One

We may hear "professional" and think of a clinical atmosphere or a distant and aloof therapist. Nothing could be further from the truth. Professionalism doesn't mean acting stuffy or keeping our clients at arms' length. It simply means that, when we're working, our focus is our clients. We pay attention to them, we're sensitive to their vulnerability. Being professional is just an educated way of being kind.

The way that we demonstrate this kindness is by keeping safe boundaries. Boundaries* are the way we define our relationships as professional and therefore, safe. For instance, not asking a client for a date or not giving advice about medical issues would be part of good boundaries—boundaries are about keeping things *out* as much as they are about keeping things in. (An example of things kept in would be information about the client.) Boundaries clarify what will happen between client and practitioner. A casual attitude toward boundaries can jar clients and make them uneasy. Solid boundaries are a comfort.

Usually when clients complain about an experience they had with a practitioner, their complaint is not about technique or knowledge of anatomy. They say, "She talked about her boyfriend the whole hour," or "She wanted to know more about my personal life than I wanted to tell her," or "I felt nervous going to a bodyworker who works out of a bedroom in his house."

---

*For definition, see page 227.

As much as we want to be respectful and kind, many manual therapists* haven't been trained in either the value or the how-to's of maintaining professional boundaries. When we have made mistakes with clients, it has been mostly from lack of education and awareness. Some of us have learned through painful experience. A colleague who was trained in working with clients' emotional issues but not taught to create safe boundaries said:

> A couple of years into my practice, I realized that it was a mess. Clients became friends, friends became clients and I was putting a good deal of energy into sorting it out. Plus, I began to realize that the client's work never went as deep once we had crossed into being social. When I became clearer with boundaries, my work became easier and my clients were able to go to a deeper level.

Our profession is still young. We're learning that being a good practitioner is more than just knowing technique and that the therapeutic relationship requires more than just friendliness and warmth. For clients to relax and drop their guard, they need the security and safety of sturdy professional boundaries.

Creating Safety

A safe environment is predictable, consistent and focused on our clients. Clients know what the contract* is and what service is to be provided for what fee. Outside that agreement, they are free to concentrate on their own process without tending to our needs. It's an environment in which the client doesn't

---

*For definitions, see pages 228 & 229.

feel judged, criticized or sized up as either a potential buddy or potential sexual partner.

It may sound obvious, yet keeping the boundaries of a session really crisp isn't easy. To create an ideal, immaculately safe session we would have to eliminate all the times we worked with friends, did trades, talked about ourselves unnecessarily, complained about anything in our lives, talked about other clients or offered counseling, nutritional advice or any unasked-for words of wisdom. For starters.

We would have to be ready on time with a clean, quiet, private space that's free from interruption. We wouldn't promise results we couldn't deliver, give an inflated idea of our skills, become chummy with clients or say words that cause a client to tighten up instead of taking a deep breath and letting go.

Keeping good boundaries is a little like steering a car—there's constant correction. Just when we think we've got it, we hit a bump. It's not a question of *whether* we make mistakes: we're bound to make mistakes. It's a question of knowing when we've made mistakes and knowing what to do about them.

> A colleague who often gave advice to an unhappily-married client realized that he was in over his head. He told the client he'd be glad to be just a sympathetic ear for her, but if she wanted to work on changing her relationship with her husband, he would help her find a good marriage counselor.

> A bodyworker told me that when he talks too much during a session, he literally gets a bad

taste in his mouth. That's the way he knows he needs to be quiet and listen to his client.

Before and after vacations, boundaries can become haphazard. Following some time off, a colleague realized she was dragging in just a few minutes late to all her sessions. Once she noticed what she was doing, she was able to make extra efforts to be on time.

All professionals make boundary mistakes. However, manual therapists may need to be even more careful than other professionals—just by touching people we have already crossed accepted cultural norms.

The Need for Safety

We can take the intimacy of our work for granted and forget how scary and potentially intrusive our touch may be for clients. We live in a culture in which touch is often experienced as leading to seduction or violence. Yet our profession asks us to put our hands on strangers who are often naked or only partially clothed. In a society obsessed with being trim and blemish-free, we ask people to reveal their less-than-perfect bodies. And then we wonder why some clients have a hard time relaxing?

We are an unknown to much of the public. They may associate our work with "massage parlors." They may be frightened by the differentness of our work and wary of our lack of medical credentials. They may be afraid that we will hurt them or make them feel worse. It's up to us to define the situation as safe. It's up to us to show that we are serious about what we do and concerned about their welfare.

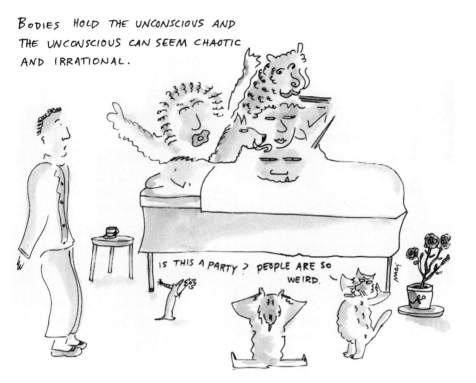

BODIES HOLD THE UNCONSCIOUS AND
THE UNCONSCIOUS CAN SEEM CHAOTIC
AND IRRATIONAL.

IS THIS A PARTY? PEOPLE ARE SO WEIRD.

The Body And the Unconscious

As best we can, we need to provide an environment that reassures clients that they are safe. Touch can stir up long-buried feelings and memories that clients find both surprising and frightening. Bodies hold the unconscious and the unconscious can seem chaotic and irrational.

Growing up in even the most caring of families, as children, we learn to hold back feelings that we think we shouldn't have or to censor the aspects of ourselves that make the people around us uncomfortable. We shut away memories that threaten to overwhelm us. When we hold back feelings, aspects of ourselves

15

or memories, we literally hold them back with our muscles. What is held back can get locked into our tissue. This is true whether the holding was last week or decades ago. When we are touched, those memories and feelings may emerge. Many of us know this from experience:

> A massage therapist loosens a client's shoulders and suddenly, the client remembers how angry she was at her boss that week.

> A sixty-year-old structural integration client says he doesn't remember having any old injuries, but when the practitioner works with his ankle, it's as if he hit the play button of a tape recorder. The client recalls a memory of falling out of a tree and spraining his ankle when he was ten. He remembers the incident as if it were yesterday—details of what happened, how his father reacted, how scared he felt.

> A movement education client cries as subtle shifts in her pelvis reawaken the long-buried nightmare of the months she spent in a punitive home for unwed mothers twenty years earlier.

Clients bring all of their held-back memories and feelings to the table. Those feelings aren't conscious and they will not necessarily come into consciousness during a session. Nevertheless, we want to respect the fact that being touched can help a client access potentially scary and unpleasant material. Because of that, we need to provide a safe and comforting emotional atmosphere.

Power and Responsibility

The dynamics of the client/practitioner relationship are more complex than many of us realize. Our clients automatically give us more power than they would, for instance, if they met us on the street. Because of that power imbalance, we need to maintain secure boundaries. For practitioners, the therapeutic relationship* brings with it built-in authority and responsibilities.

Our clients come to us in pain or in need of help. Just by showing up at our offices, they make themselves vulnerable. They are hurting and we are the authority. Even though they may not be conscious of it, we can become a doctor/parent figure in their eyes. Our responsibility is to meet that vulnerability with respect and kindness.

Common Misconceptions

Many practitioners haven't been trained in the dynamics of the therapeutic relationship, and therefore don't understand the ways the unconscious influences our work. They may not understand the reasons boundaries are necessary for a client's security. Left to their own devices, many practitioners have simply done their best, piecing together their own idea of professional conduct. Here are some common misconceptions, born out of understandable confusion, that have not served us well:

Misconception #1: "I want to be natural with my clients."
This argument against keeping appropriate boundaries comes in many forms: "I want to be authentic with my clients;" "I don't want to put myself above my clients." Behind these arguments, there are compassionate concepts of equality and a desire not to see ourselves as superior. Although we're not

---
*For definition, see page 229.

personally superior to our clients, as professionals, we are taking on a special role with them. It's a role that requires us, for their own good, to be careful what we reveal about ourselves.

Sharing personal information with clients can put them in the position of having to take care of us in the way that friends tend to each other. At the least, it takes attention away from the reason they are there—to have *us* pay attention to *their* needs. It's misguided to think that behaving with clients as we do with friends is therapeutic for clients. We might, for instance, complain about our love lives to a client under the rationale of being real. While we may have good intentions, hearing about our personal concerns or knowing about our personal lives is not usually helpful to the client.

Authenticity is reassuring when we are down-to-earth in our presentation of ourselves, when we don't mystify what we are doing or pretend to be all-knowing. It can be healing to allow clients to see the compassion we feel towards them. We can, for instance, let clients see that their stories have touched us; we can become tearful with clients about *their* concerns but not our own.

Boundaries aren't elitist. Quite the opposite. A safe and clear relationship between practitioner and client keeps the focus where it needs to be—on the client.

Misconception #2: "I'll just use my common sense."
We may think that professionalism is just common sense, but it's not that simple. Making good judgments doesn't come naturally. After we've practiced long enough, we can begin to look and feel like "naturals," but it's never the same as just being ourselves or only using common sense.

Without guidelines, our boundary and ethics decisions are likely to be based on a hodgepodge of conflicting influences. We are affected by what our upbringing has taught us about pain, dependency, sex and intimacy. We're swayed by our own biases and prejudices. Our judgment can be clouded by our egos and by the all-too-human need to be in control, right or important. Or we may imitate mentors and teachers who didn't themselves understand the need for good boundaries. We may rely on advice from our friends or partners. And, when in doubt, we may throw in a random piece of wisdom from the latest self-help book we read.

Making good judgment calls takes knowing ourselves and working through our issues; that's the difficult part. We can know in our heads the "right" thing to do, and still not do it. If, for instance, our own boundaries have been violated as children—sexually, psychologically or physically—then what comes "naturally" to us may still be off-kilter.

Even if we have had no significant childhood trauma, we bring to our work all our unresolved wounds. We all have blind spots that interfere with our effectiveness. We have patches in our behavior where we don't make sense, see the obvious or act rationally. We deny, rationalize and project the things we dislike about ourselves onto other people. It's just a part of being human.

> A colleague gained unwanted weight, and for the next couple of months found himself mentally judging his overweight clients. He finally realized what he was doing and why, and was able to stop his negative reactions.

A massage therapist with a history of sexual abuse routinely used to overlap her social life and her professional life, urging people she found attractive to come to her for massage, for instance. At the time, she didn't see the connection between the boundary confusion of her abuse and the boundary confusion she played out in her practice.

We all have blind spots and we're all imperfect. Good boundaries are too crucial to leave to our unreliable common sense.

Misconception #3: "I've learned technique and that's all I need to know."
Until recently, medical schools focused on teaching anatomy and technique, as if the relationship with the patient didn't matter. Perhaps, without thinking, we have used that attitude as a model. Until recently, many of our own schools have put the emphasis on anatomy and technique—ignoring the importance of relationship dynamics. While that omission is understandable, practitioners who were taught only anatomy and technique may continue to believe that's all that matters.

Fortunately, many massage and manual therapy schools (along with many medical schools) have added courses on boundaries, ethics, transference* and the importance of a healing alliance between practitioner and client. We are giving up the old idea of teaching the manual therapies as if people were just a mass of muscles to be manipulated.

Doctors would benefit from maintaining better boundaries—how often are they on time for appointments? As manual therapists, we may need to pay even more attention to boundaries than doctors do. In going to a doctor, people don't

---

*For definition, see page 230.

expect to let go and have a blissful, transcendent experience. But when people come to us, they are hoping to be able to drop their defenses. They want to leave feeling more centered, more alive, more themselves. Setting the stage for that experience requires a good deal more education and training than just learning the name of the erector spinae. No exotic technique by itself will ensure that a client will trust us. (Impeccable boundaries won't ensure trust either, but they will improve the odds.)

How people heal is a mystery. Humans are a complicated mix of psyche, spirit, body and emotions and we can't even know where one of those elements stops and another starts. We can learn a hundred new techniques and still not understand why people hurt. But we can create an atmosphere within which we and our clients can explore the mystery.

Misconception #4: "I have needs too."

> A massage therapist who canceled a session at the last minute to attend to personal business didn't appreciate why her client, a woman in pain who had been looking forward to her session, got so upset. The therapist told me, "My clients have to understand that I have needs too."

Of course the massage therapist has personal needs—we all do. But it's inappropriate to bring them into the professional setting. We're there to focus on our clients' needs, which means putting our personal lives aside during a session. Although we can't avoid the occasional intrusion of a personal situation into our work, we have to realize that *professional* means "the show must go on" and, when it cannot, we let our clients down. (We can consider offering a free session when we are forced to cancel without sufficient notice.)

Along with being sensitive to clients' discomfort, being professional means that we can expect our clients to treat us as professionals and not cause *us* discomfort. It's perfectly kosher, and even desirable, to be concerned with our *professional* needs. We have a legitimate need to be competent and skilled at our work, and to be treated as serious professionals whose clients respect our time and fees. For instance, we can expect our clients to pay at each session and to give adequate cancellation notice.

Sometimes new practitioners have difficulty setting limits. They may allow clients to cancel at the last minute without paying for the session, for example, or give a full session to clients who arrive twenty minutes late. They allow clients to take advantage of them, which can lead to resentment on their part and confusion on the part of the client.

Professional boundaries define the therapeutic relationship as having limits and standards that both practitioner and client are to respect. They benefit both parties by helping us feel more secure in what is a uniquely intimate situation.

Misconception #5: "My connection with my clients is through the healing energy in my hands."
That's a good start—but is it enough? This work is intuitive and there can be an energetic relationship with our clients that's hard to define. But that isn't all there is to it. If we get too caught up in the mystery of our work, we can overlook our clients' basic needs. We can gaze into the distance with misty eyes and speak of our magical connection with our clients, but

if that's our only focus, our clients will be wondering why the room is so cold, why we were ten minutes late and why we won't stop talking about our new car.

Nothing is wrong with having needs of our own or wanting to be natural with our clients. Nothing is wrong with sensing the magic in the connections we make with our clients. But, if we're not careful, those attitudes can become rationales for unprofessional behavior.

Coming of Age

Our profession is coming of age, establishing its own identity. We're rightfully concerned about our public image. Paying attention to the details of professional boundaries is the way we can elevate our status as health care professionals.

Attention to boundaries is also the key to a smoothly running practice. When we create a safe environment, our clients settle in and go deeper. Our work lives flow more smoothly. We have more satisfied clients who come back and who tell their friends about us. We have fewer difficult clients and more clients who leave our offices with a lighter heart and a lighter step.

We become massage therapists, bodyworkers and movement teachers because of our compassion, but compassion needs the structure of good professional boundaries. To really serve our clients, we need not merely good hearts, but educated hearts.

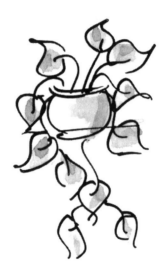

Boundaries: Protective Circles

✖

Chapter Two

The work of the manual therapies is unusual and sometimes intrusive. Just the fact that we touch people goes beyond cultural norms about personal boundaries. What we do is unfamiliar to much of the public and its intimacy can stir up deep emotional associations. How do we make this potentially confusing and highly charged situation safe for our clients and for ourselves?

Boundaries are the heart of how we protect both ourselves and our clients. A boundary is like a protective circle drawn around ourselves and our clients: it defines what goes on within that circle and the ways practitioners and their clients will and will not treat each other.

Defining Boundaries

Boundaries clarify each person's limits and expectations. The concept sounds simple. The agreement is that the client will come to us for massage therapy, bodywork or movement education. We will do what we are trained to do and what we have contracted to do. The client will pay us an agreed-upon amount or complete a prearranged trade. The agreement may sound simple, but it can be easy to lose our focus and overstep boundaries.

We may decide, for instance, that we have valuable advice to offer—how to save a marriage, what vitamins to take or which spiritual retreat would best suit the client. Or we may want to get to know the client socially. We need to remember what we have contracted to do. What is our role in the therapeutic relationship?

Roles

Taking on a role doesn't mean we are pretending. Rather, it means that we have agreed to behave in certain ways during our interactions with that client. The therapeutic relationship is determined by what we've been trained to do and by what the client is paying us to do. We may have training in clinical psychology, for instance, but if clients are coming to us for acupressure, we don't take on the role of psychological counselor.

We always have two roles with our clients: the broader role is that of the professional and the second is the one defined by our specific training—massage therapist or Feldenkrais teacher or Trager practitioner and so on. In any manual therapy training, we should learn both.

Our training should teach us how to take a professional stance. It should teach us, for instance, how to keep our personal lives, opinions and needs out of our sessions. We should also learn how professionals are to be treated and that we have the right to be treated as professionals.

During training we also begin to identify with our chosen fields and with other people who do what we are learning to do—often taking on role models or following the teachings of significant leaders in our field. We also learn both the spoken rules and ethics and the unspoken rules that go with being a certain kind of practitioner. In this way we begin to make the shift from thinking of ourselves as bottle washers (or whatever we were doing before our manual therapy training) to thinking of ourselves as massage therapists, Alexander teachers, Zero Balancers, Reiki masters, etc.

Learning to be at ease with those two roles—as a professional and as a certain type of practitioner—takes time. Those whose training was relatively short may have missed out on this vital part of their education and need to fill that gap another way. We can learn massage strokes in a weekend, but it takes a much longer time to ease into a solid sense of ourselves as professional manual therapists.

Most Common Boundary Mistakes

If we stuck with our appropriate roles, we wouldn't have as much trouble with boundaries. But as a profession, the field of manual therapy is still relatively new. We're still defining our place in the larger scheme of things, still clarifying what our role in health care is. We're also human and make mistakes.

There are common areas of boundary confusion, where staying in bounds sometimes requires us to walk a fine line. Are we giving psychological counseling when we reassure a depressed client? Are we giving medical advice when we suggest that a client doesn't need an orthotic device (shoe lift) anymore? When are we overstepping the friendship line? What is too much information about ourselves to give a client?

The practitioner who thinks he or she never violates boundaries has cause for concern. If we understand boundaries and pay close attention to what we're doing, we know that we often make errors—usually small ones that we can easily adjust. We will never arrive at perfection; we have to keep learning and correcting our errors. The challenge is to be aware of boundaries and to value them, yet be tolerant of our imperfection. Since our mistakes are usually at the client's expense, we don't want to be too tolerant.

Most experienced practitioners will recognize some, or perhaps much, of their behavior in the don't-do-this column. The fact that, over the years, we constantly made the kinds of mistakes discussed in this chapter doesn't mean it's time to abandon our office and go work in a donut shop. For one thing, practicing the manual therapies is difficult and most of us have received little information or education in the area of boundaries. Most of us have felt, and perhaps rightly so, that just by coming to work with our shirt tails tucked in, providing clean sheets and not sleeping with our clients, we've been professional. For another thing, giving advice or having tea with clients doesn't mean we're unfit practitioners: we can make those mistakes and still be good professionals who have helped many people. However, if we want to jump to another level, if what we want is to achieve a level of *mastery* in our work, taking the time and trouble to learn to maintain crisp boundaries is the place to start. It can make our work lives simpler and easier, and our work deeper and more satisfying.

Clients' Complaints
Clients' complaints about practitioners typically fall into two categories:

(1)   Going beyond the boundaries of our expertise—promising too much, giving advice or counseling outside our level of training.

(2)   Blurring the line between our social and professional roles—using the client to meet

28

our personal social needs. This can be as
subtle as chatting about our own lives
during a session or as complicated as
turning clients into lovers.

The first boundary mistake, going beyond our expertise, often
stems from professional insecurity. The second one, making
our interactions with clients into social events, often comes
from our isolation and/or boredom. These aren't just individual
issues of insecurity or isolation: being unsure of the worth of
our profession or feeling isolated in a practice are problems
many practitioners have in common.

Given the critical importance of both these issues, they will be
discussed more at length.

Going Outside Our Expertise

We go beyond the boundaries of our expertise when we make
exaggerated claims about the effects of our method or when we
behave as if we have training in areas that we do not. For instance,
we are on thin ice if we guarantee that massage will help a client's
blood pressure. Likewise, if we tell clients what foods to eat or
why they should divorce their spouses, we venture into territory
for which we have no training and no contract.

The Insecurity of "The Total Healer"

When I completed my training as a Certified Rolfer, there was
hardly any physical or emotional condition that I didn't think
I could fix. From hemorrhoids to schizophrenia—I thought
Rolfing could heal it. I don't think that kind of grandiosity is
limited just to Rolfers. Many practitioners display it, often
when just out of school and inexperienced.

For one thing, most of us become practitioners of a certain method because we're impressed by the effect it had on us. We've often seen a wide range of symptoms clear up— sometimes ones seemingly unrelated to the mode of treatment. Also, during our training, our teachers tell us stories of miraculous healings. We forget that the stories we hear are select, the most dramatic stories from those teachers' years of experience.

Even though our teachers may be very clear about the limits of what our work can achieve, we may leave our training with unrealistic expectations. We may begin to think that our everyday work life should be filled with amazing cures—people casting canes and crutches aside, diabetics throwing away their insulin, depressives no longer needing medication. All of these have indeed occurred as a result of effective bodywork—but not routinely, and there are no guarantees.

There is also, along with these elevated expectations, our professional insecurity. On a personal level, particularly when we are just out of school, we are unsure of ourselves. Deep down we may think we have no business doing this work. We may think, "What on earth do I have to offer people? Surely someone will notice that I don't know what I'm doing."

In addition, as a profession, manual therapists are insecure. We don't live in a culture where ads on the bus read "Got aches and pains? Consult your bodyworker first." The benefits of our work are becoming more widely known, but many people still don't know how it can help them. For the most part, the manual therapies are still unacknowledged by a culture accustomed to a traditional medical viewpoint. For many of us, there is a vast gap between what we know to be the value of our work and the value given to it by most of the public. Sometimes in our frustration with the lack of recognition, we swing the other way and promise too much.

Bragging, promising too much, overinflating the merits of our brand of work are all signs of insecurity, as is putting down other methodologies. Our motivations for becoming manual therapists are complex, but generally, we have a desire to help people in pain. It's difficult to just tell them the simple truth— to say to someone in acute suffering, "Maybe this will help and maybe it won't. You might even feel worse before you feel better." It's even harder to say, "I don't have enough training (or skill) to help you. Let me refer you to a more advanced practitioner (or another kind of health professional)."

The reasons for pain are complex and multilayered. No matter how knowledgeable we are, there is much we don't know. Our methods, no matter how beneficial, can only do so much. Rather than face the fact that there are limits to what we can do, we begin to lean on an inflated idea of our own abilities and the benefits of our work. (This can be true of the medical profession as well.)

The Weekend Workshop Syndrome

Many of us are constantly looking for ways to advance our knowledge of ourselves and our work. We take workshops to add new techniques to our repertoire; we attend seminars that help us with personal discovery and spiritual growth.

Weekend workshops can re-energize us and give us new ideas and techniques to explore. Personal growth workshops can free us to have healthier relationships with our clients. But these short courses can also give fresh meaning to the phrase, "A little knowledge is a dangerous thing." Sometimes weekend workshops produce "instant experts." I've seen people with a weekend workshop or two under their belts doing cervical adjustments, holding forth on neurological problems or claiming to understand the causes of cancer. These are dangerous presumptions of expertise.

It's also not appropriate to set ourselves up as spiritual advisers. It might be offensive to our clients. Sandy Fritz, owner of Health Enrichment Center in Michigan and author of massage therapy textbooks, teaches her students how to identify clients with spiritual issues. For instance, when clients talk about their lives being empty or meaningless, what practitioners can do is help clients see that these are spiritual issues, but not offer recommendations or advice. We could say, "Your questions strike me as involving spirituality," or "Your recent conversations have sounded as if you're moving toward an important realization." If we think we have had a spiritual awakening, rather than preaching or giving our clients "The Answer," we can use our spirituality to be kinder to them.

The real answer is that the revelation or new technique that meant so much to us on Saturday afternoon probably isn't appropriate for our Monday morning client. And taking a weekend workshop in cranial sacral work, for instance, doesn't qualify us as cranial experts—considering that cranial osteopaths generally have had at least 10,000 hours of study and hands-on practice before they ever start to work with the public.

Little Docs

Manual therapists' technical skills have advanced rapidly over the past ten years. Paralleling those advances is increasing confusion about our ability to handle medical situations.

> I recently overheard bodyworkers discussing how to handle someone's prospective client who had a rare disorder that affected her thoracic spine. All kinds of advice was given about which vertebra to work with, which to avoid and how to help her. Everyone's intentions were clearly good, but all these suggestions came from practitioners who had never seen the client and knew nothing of her history, nor the severity of her problem. Nor did any of them have special training to work with this rare disorder.

> Finally, a teacher who had been standing aside weighed in with the obvious point that we should never see a client with such a complicated medical problem without consulting her doctor. He also said that he personally would not treat this client under any circumstances because it was beyond his level of expertise.

Many of the practitioners interviewed for this book expressed concern about practitioners who treat medical issues without sufficient training and/or without consultation with the client's doctor, chiropractor, naturopath, etc. Such boundary violations can be as simple as giving advice that's traditionally in the medical realm—such as advising a client to give up an ankle brace or to cut back on medication. Or they can be as dangerous as working with a serious medical condition without input from the appropriate medical practitioner. There are ethical considerations that will be further explored in Chapter Five on Ethics.

If we give an opinion, we need to identify it as a personal opinion if it doesn't come from our training. And we need to take care how we state an opinion. "I've known some people who used vitamin C for colds and got good results" is safer to say than "You should take vitamin C."

But beyond a concern for staying out of legal hot water, we want to honor the dictum, "First, do no harm." Although we can sometimes help a client who hasn't been helped by the usual medical regimen of drugs or surgery, that doesn't mean that we can hang out a shingle that reads "The Doctor is In." Most clients already give us more authority than is rightfully ours. It's up to us to stay honest and within the bounds of what we know.

The Power of Not Knowing

It's important not to be afraid to say "I don't know." It's a respectable answer. When a client asks me a medical question, such as how to treat a sprain, I still hold my breath when I answer, "I don't know—I'm not trained in that area." Rather than the reaction I fear ("You don't know everything? Then why am I here?"), clients simply shrug and go on to the next topic.

Not having to know everything is very freeing and our clients appreciate the honesty of an "I don't know." It educates them about what we do know. Showing our clients that we honor our limits helps them trust us.

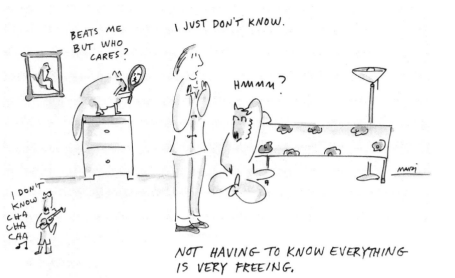

NOT HAVING TO KNOW EVERYTHING IS VERY FREEING.

Feeling that we have to *always* know what's going on can make our work stressful and stifle our curiosity. We'll find ourselves falling back on rote answers. "Anger is in the shoulders." "The way to work with this kind of knee is to do X." Having to know can make us miss out on what's going on right here, right now— in front of us, with this client.

Psychology and Emotions

The most complex judgment calls about boundaries are in the realm of the emotional and psychological. When are we being friendly and when are we making a mistake by acting like amateur psychotherapists? As practitioners, it's appropriate to be sensitive to our clients and supportive of them. It's important to get to know them. Often, the more we know of their lives and concerns, the more we can help them. (Although we need to respect the privacy of clients who don't want to reveal their personal lives.)

When are we inappropriately stepping into the role of psychotherapist? Actually we usually don't so much *step* into the role as stumble into it. Before we know it, we've stumbled and slid into giving advice or counseling when we don't really have the training. Anytime anything we do goes beyond good listening, we're probably heading down the wrong road.

Counseling is more than just common sense. The difficult part of being a good counselor or psychotherapist is learning to be aware of and skillfully deal with transference* and countertransference* issues—all the unconscious interpersonal reactions that both we and the client bring to a session. (Transference and countertransference are discussed more in Chapter Three). Psychotherapists spend years in supervision learning to identify and handle their client's transference and their own countertransference. Similarly, practitioners of bodywork methods that access deep emotional issues often spend years in ongoing supervision before they are considered skilled enough to become full-fledged practitioners.

Although most of us don't have training in psychology, and probably know better than to play psychotherapists, we can still fall into the trap of naively giving advice about personal matters. Our motivation is good: we want to help the client. After all, we have our accumulated personal experience, we've read books and maybe we've been in therapy ourselves. We may have had emotional openings that were useful or even profound. We care about our clients; we see their unhappiness and want to share our experiences and philosophies with them.

Appropriate Helping
Practitioners who try to act like counselors are often clumsy—

---

*For definitions, see pages 228 & 230.

doing things that a good therapist wouldn't do, such as giving advice, confronting clients bluntly, making hasty interpretations. Even if we have training in these areas, we must look at the reason the client has come to us. If he comes to us for a sore lower back, it's not our business to tell him that he's angry at his boss.

So what do we do when we have good reason to believe that a client's bad back *may be* aggravated by his inability to stand up to his boss? What do we do when we think that if a client could just let go of that holding behind the right scapula, most of his pain would disappear? Appropriate intervention would be to say, "Notice how tense your back gets when you talk about your boss." Or, "There's a tight place behind your left shoulder blade that always seems to be there." As manual therapists, our expertise comes from what we see in clients' bodies and what we feel under our hands. That information is what we have to offer our clients. Sharing it with them can be valuable and healing.

Listening

The other action we can take—and often it is the best response—is to just listen. We forget how powerful it is to have someone simply listen. As practitioners, we can feel tempted to take charge when someone sounds confused. We can be tempted to give advice or to share an experience from our lives that seems similar to the client's issue. It's natural to want to "do something" when we see another's distress.

Listening to the client's words and the client's body beneath our hands is the most vital skill we have. When we're listening and tuned in, there's a flow and a resonance with the client that opens the door for healing to happen, with nothing more said.

Forcing Emotional Release

Physically pushing clients towards emotional release can be even more invasive and harmful than pressuring them verbally. For one thing, we're making big assumptions when we think we know what that tight place in the client's back is holding, and we think we know when and how to release it. We're also assuming that forcing an area open will somehow be healing. Forcing a release is disrespectful and violates the client's vulnerability. It makes the practitioner the "powerful" one and the client the passive one who is acted upon; it can even re-traumatize an already traumatized client.

Referrals

If someone is suicidal or very depressed or if someone is continuously agitated or confused, we need to refer them to a mental health professional. Most of the situations we deal with aren't that cut and dried, however. To help us sort out where our responsibilities are, we need to get good supervision* from a more experienced practitioner.

Confusing Professional with Social

The other major area of boundary confusion is losing the distinction between our professional lives and our social lives. This can be such a touchy subject for bodyworkers. Many believe that making strict rules about socializing is going too far. What's wrong with sharing something about ourselves with our clients during a session? What's wrong with a friendly cup of tea? Maybe nothing is—but these actions risk interfering with how clients receive our work.

In a professional relationship, the total focus is on the well-being of the client. Putting clients in the role of friends or

---

*For definition, see page 229.

confidantes dilutes that focus and short-changes them as clients. Clients need to see us as someone who is there for them. They need *not* to have to take care of us, *not* to know about our aches and pains, our emotional conflicts, our unresolved issues. The more we muddy the waters between the social and the professional, the more likely we are to do or say something that will interfere with having a professional, healing relationship.

> A female bodyworker working with a male client used his sessions to lament the woes of her divorce and the problems of being single. This was confusing to the client—he interpreted her personal revelations to mean that she wanted a more social or romantic relationship with him. When he asked her out, however, she refused him. He ended up feeling hurt and rejected and stopped going to her as a bodyworker.

In the above example, the client ended up feeling wounded by a relationship that should have been therapeutic. We cheat our clients when we put the focus on ourselves, when we ask them to listen to us and take care of us. We also can lose clients that way.

A common complaint about manual therapists is that we talk too much about ourselves during a session. Clients will rarely ask us to be quiet. They won't say, "I can't take another minute of your talking about your cat." Clients are both too polite and too much under the influence of the power imbalance that's inherent in the relationship.

Sometimes clients will ask us personal questions. To answer the client appropriately, we first need to understand the reason the client is asking the question. Otherwise, we may tend to either give out more information than they need or shut them out in an abrupt way. A client asking, "Are you married?" could be asking if we can understand the difficulty he is having with his spouse. Or he could be asking if we are available for a date. These are two different scenarios that would have two different responses. In the first instance, we could say, "I understand how hard it is to keep clear communication with your partner." Whether or not we would reveal our marital status is a judgment call in that instance. If, on the other hand, we think a client wants to ask us out, we could tell the client we don't give out personal information or we could simply stop the questions by saying that we're not available.

There are other reasons clients may ask us personal questions: some clients, especially women, feel uncomfortable or impolite if the focus of the session is entirely on them. We need to let such clients know that the session is their time and that it's fine for them to relax and concentrate only on the work we are doing and on their own concerns.

To stay focused on the client, we need to appreciate the client's motivation for asking us the question. We might even say, "I'll be willing to answer that but first, I'm curious why you're asking. How would it help you to know that?" Our work should be client-centered and we always want to turn the spotlight back on them—but in a friendly way. We don't want to carry this idea to silly extremes:

> A practitioner who had newly-learned the technique of turning the question back on the

client showed up at his office one morning with his foot in a cast. When his first client asked, "How did you break your foot?" his response was "How do you *think* I broke my foot?"

Such responses can feel withholding or patronizing to a client. Our goal is always to show respect for the client. We want to find a balance between the above response and giving the client a fifteen minute monologue about our broken foot. Again, what we want to discern and respond to is the reason the client is asking. A client inquiring about a practitioner's broken foot could be wondering if the wounded practitioner can now more readily identify with her pain or she may be asking, "Even though you are injured, can you still help me today?" Responding appropriately is much more complex than it looks and needs to be thoughtful, rather than automatic.

Is It Really Friendship?

"But I become friends with my clients," we protest. We may be on friendly terms with our clients, but are they really like our friends? Do we have friends who come to see us and immediately throw off their clothes and describe all their ailments and fears? Funny friends.

Personal friends put up with our lapses and our flaws; they listen patiently while we go on for ten minutes about what somebody said to us and what we said back. They forgive us when we act like jerks or hurt their feelings. Friends aren't paying us.

Once someone becomes a client, we need to always be aware of our therapeutic role, both in and out of a session. When we find ourselves in a social situation with a client or even bumping into one on the street, we want to remain mindful of our responsibility toward that person. We want to take care not to reveal anything about ourselves that might detract from the person's capacity to feel safe with us. Clients don't need to know that we are tired, unhappy about the weather, etc. Even the smallest personal revelation can make a vulnerable client doubt our capabilities or put the client into a care-taking role. In casual encounters, keep the conversation light and the focus on the client. (And, of course, don't bring up or talk about anything related to the client's sessions.) Not many clients will complain if they're the focus of our interactions—most people won't even notice; they'll just appreciate the attention.

Sexual Energy

There's another reason to avoid the temptation to socialize with our clients. Let's be honest—when the wish to socialize is there, isn't it sometimes because we're attracted to that client? Perhaps the client has a crush on us that we're enjoying. Dating a client or flirting with a client isn't good for the client, and it's bad for the practitioner's reputation. We don't want to even start moving in that direction.

The Loneliness of Our Work

Alexander instructor Vivien Schapera thinks we resist the idea of separating our business life from our social life because we don't want to face the essential loneliness of our work.

She notes that we have a unique role in the community: we're not doctors or therapists; we're more like peers, but we are also held in esteem and seen as special. Because we have a certain status and are also privy to confidential information, we have a responsibility to our clients. With people who are or have been our clients, we must always remain, to some extent, aware of our role. We always have to ask ourselves whether our behavior with clients is beneficial to them. We can never truly relax or "let our hair down." We can't expect them to ever see who we are in the same way that a non-client would. Being a "healer" in a community can be a lonely responsibility.

Many of us work by ourselves, even out of our homes. There isn't the constant opportunity for social interaction that we would have working in most jobs. Because we don't have buddies we can meet over the water cooler to unload the day-to-day trivia and drama of our lives, we can be tempted to use our clients as a captive audience.

Our work is stressful, which makes our isolation harder to tolerate. Hopefully, we're dealing with satisfied customers who leave smiling and relaxed, but we're basically up to our elbows in other people's pain, discomfort and unhappiness. We hear their secrets. We sometimes know things about them that even people who live with them don't know. Sometimes we feel unable to help them. These are hard things to carry within ourselves.

Once we recognize the loneliness of our position and the responsibilities that go with it, we can take steps to make our work lives easier. We can create our own support groups and helpers. We can find mentors and seek out supervision. We can find ways to get satisfaction from the work we do without using our clients' sessions to meet our social needs.

Boredom
Any work can become routine and boring. The two hundred and fiftieth time we effleurage an arm may not be as interesting as the first ten.

During a workshop for massage therapy students, I was surprised to hear that one of their main complaints was clients who talked during their massage. The students were trying to concentrate on remembering what to do and were distracted by a talking client. They had a hard time believing that, in a few months, when they were more familiar with techniques, they might occasionally get bored and may *want* their clients to entertain them by talking.

We have to find additional ways to make our work life stimulating and interesting. True, some clients may actually want to talk with us and that can be an important part of the work. Talking may relieve their tension; the issues they bring up may, whether they know it or not, be key to their opening to the work. But, we should always take our cues from the client, and not initiate idle conversation or talk about our own lives and opinions.

Boundaries Aren't Barriers

Boundaries aren't barriers between practitioner and client. They're not intended to keep clients at arms' length or to allow practitioners to act superior. Every relationship in our lives has boundaries. They tell us what to expect and what's appropriate in a particular situation. Boundaries are a natural part of everyone's world.

Boundaries help keep us within the limits of our training. They keep our egos and our insecurities out of our sessions, and they keep us honest. Boundaries help us show the best of ourselves. To be skillful and compassionate with clients, we start by attending to boundaries.

Client/Practitioner Dynamics: The Power Imbalance

❌

Chapter Three

The minute we take on a client, we acquire a responsibility toward that person. The relationship is lopsided and unequal and it is likely to continue that way for as long as we know him. In the client's eyes, the practitioner has special authority and power and that perception may churn up strong unconscious feelings. Because of that, we have an obligation to create a safe space for our clients.

The intimacy of the situation may bring up unconscious issues for the client—and for us. That holds true even if our work is not deep or emotionally-oriented.* In what other kind of relationship is one person clothed and the other not, one person putting nurturing hands on a relatively passive other? Parent/child? Doctor/patient? Lovers? Clients often see us as more than we really are.

Clients will tell us things that they wouldn't ordinarily tell a virtual stranger. They'll ask our advice on matters we may know nothing about. Some of them will think we're warm and loving, while others will watch us with a wary eye.

Psychotherapists call this transference—clients respond to us with feelings and attitudes that were originally associated with important people (parents, siblings, etc.) from childhood. They transfer those feelings to us. The feelings can be positive or negative; they can be idealized fantasies about the parent they

---

*For definition, see page 228.

never had or feelings of mistrust for all parental figures. Transference is an unconscious process.

Actually, we all "do transference" all the time; for instance, we may over-react to a boyfriend's teasing because a father's critical attitude was hurtful, or feel especially connected to a friend who looks and acts like an adored mother. But, in a manual therapy session, the unconscious may be more actively involved than in our everyday life. Often, both client and practitioner enter into an altered state; as a result, we sink beneath our rational minds and are more in contact with our unconscious.

In order to serve our clients well, we have to understand the effects of transference. For one thing, we need to understand that taking on the role of practitioner gives us an added authority—how we behave with clients and the words we say will carry extra weight. Statements that sound judgmental will sink in deeper than if they were, for instance, said by someone with whom the client was talking at a meeting. Compassionate words from a practitioner can have an equally strong positive effect. We need to take care what we say to clients:

> At the end of a session, a practitioner was taking another look at the client's body, evaluating the effects of his work on the client's tension and knots. Not pleased with how the client had progressed and absorbed in judgments of his own skill, he exclaimed, "Oh, damn!" How do you think the client felt?

> Rolfing Instructor Tom Wing is a master of diplomacy. In classes, clients have to undergo the rigors of standing in their underwear while

students and teachers evaluate their structure. At such times, Tom is always aware of a client's vulnerability and chooses his words carefully. In one instance, he had just discussed a condition in which the tissue around the knees is bunched up, known colloquially as "pineapple knees." As it happened, the next client to be evaluated was a woman who had such knees. Wanting to alert the class to this but not wanting to offend the client, Tom smiled and said, "Ah....the Hawaiian look." The class understood his point and the client felt complimented.

Understanding the effects of transference can help us take that extra step in being compassionate with clients. It can also help us in understanding clients' sometimes puzzling responses to us. This chapter will discuss how to work with some common client reactions—over-trust, mistrust, hostility or adoration.

When the *practitioner* transfers feelings to the client that belong in the practitioner's past, that is called "countertransference." Countertransference, like transference, is an unconscious process—we're not consciously aware of why we're responding to the client in a certain way. The picky, complaining client we can never please becomes, in our minds, our chronically complaining mother. That sweet client who thinks everything we do is wonderful becomes the ideal dad we longed for. The client who stops making appointments (even if it's because he's improved) becomes the parent who abandoned us. Problems arise when we begin to relate to the complaining client as if we were unhappy children, rather than compassionate professionals. Problems can occur when we think the sweet client is there to build our egos, rather than be helped by us. And when clients stop coming, we need to be able to understand it from a healthy perspective, not see it as rejection.

Appreciating the power of transference and countertransference is the key to understanding why we need to take care with boundaries. Without that understanding, ethical and boundary guidelines can seem like arbitrary rules, rather than necessary structure.

Transference: It's Not About *You*

"Transference" means it's not necessarily about us. Whether it's adoration or deep mistrust, it's often not really about the practitioner. (There is probably a grain of truth behind their reaction: we've done something that actually pleases or displeases them, but their response is out of proportion to the literal event.) We're mistaken if we think we really are that wonderful when clients adore us or that awful when they're mad at us. Clients may want to take care of us, please us, challenge us and/or berate us. None of these reactions are necessarily about us. The challenge for us is to keep an even keel and not be swayed by clients' responses.

The power of transference gives more weight to everything we do—both positive and negative. On the one hand, clients can idealize us. Our role as a supportive, warm person who touches them can make us the all-loving parent they wish they'd had or whom they had and lost. On the other hand, being "the authority" on whom they depend can stir up unconscious memories of negative or abusive parent figures, family members or authority figures. In that case, clients will come to us with unconscious expectations that they will be hurt in some way.

> A new client asks many questions about the practitioner's qualifications and during the bodywork, reacts strongly, pulling back at the slightest hint of discomfort.

> A man who grew up in Germany during World War II and experienced constant air raids and fear for his life enjoys massage therapy but is very "controlling"—telling the practitioner exactly where he wants work and how deep. He also has a hard time relaxing or even closing his eyes during a session and is constantly aware of small sounds from the outside.

Assuming that the practitioners in these examples provided a safe, welcoming space and presented themselves as professional and attentive, these clients weren't responding to the actual situation in front of them—the danger they were reacting to was in their past, not the present. It's not useful for us to respond with annoyance or dismay to behaviors like over-sensitivity, trying to take charge of the environment or hypervigilance. Understanding that old unconscious fears may motivate such reactions helps us respond with compassion and attentiveness.

Once clients connect with us as practitioners, transference just happens. Never mind that our clients are grown-ups and may even be older than 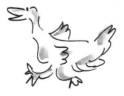 we are. Transference isn't a rational process: it's more like the way baby ducks follow after the first animal they see. It's been twenty years since I had my first Rolfing series, but if my Rolfer happened to walk by today, I would feel compelled to waddle after him, quacking and flapping.

Signs of Transference: Can't Say "No"

One sign that we've been promoted to an elevated status is that clients rarely tell us when we make them uncomfortable or when they doubt our judgment. Rarely will they say "No." If we make them too uncomfortable, they simply don't come back, sometimes not even conscious of the reason. Or they'll remain as clients but be what we call "difficult" or "resistive" clients.

When someone comes for help, they see us in a different light than if, for instance, we were to meet on the street. Clients will rarely challenge us directly; they will defer to us. There's a strong unconscious component in the therapeutic situation. This book is filled with stories of people who are generally assertive in the outside world, but who suffer without a word when they are clients.

The sense of powerlessness that usually goes with being a client is especially noticeable when the client is also a peer. I hear many stories from seasoned practitioners who have had trouble speaking up when getting work on themselves. You would think that professionals would feel comfortable asserting themselves, but because of the power of the transference, because of what happens when *they* are on the table, they may be as speechless as anyone else. If we feel powerless to question our colleagues, how must our clients feel?

- "The session ended twenty minutes earlier than usual but I didn't question it."

- "The gardener was cutting the grass with a loud lawn mower right outside the window and it was hard to focus, but I didn't say anything."

- "He expressed sexual interest in me during the session. It made me very uncomfortable, but he's such a nice guy that I didn't want to say anything."

Practitioners who tell these stories are usually bewildered or embarrassed that they didn't speak up. "I know I should have said something...," they will say apologetically.

Even in the most traumatizing situations—sexual violations—clients rarely assert themselves. There are many stories of manual therapists intentionally or unintentionally crossing a sexual boundary and then, when later confronted, protesting, "But she didn't *say* anything."

Cultural biases exaggerate the power difference between client and practitioner. The authority gap can be greater for men working with women, for a practitioner who is physically much larger than the client, for a teacher working with a student or for any practitioner who has special status in the community. It can be heightened also if we are working with a client in crisis.

> An experienced bodywork client who was having acute back spasms went to see a bodyworker who was esteemed in the community. The client said, "During the session, I felt like what she was doing wasn't right for me, but this woman is 'the best' and I didn't question her. I ended up feeling injured by her work."

Practitioners who fit any of these categories may need to take extra care to help clients feel safe. For example, many male massage therapists, particularly large men, realize that they have to take extra care to explain to clients (especially new ones) what will take place during the massage and to let clients know that they will stop the session at any time the client is uncomfortable. Although that's a good idea for all of us, for their own protection, some practitioners need to be especially alert to signs of discomfort in clients.

Signs of Transference: The Captive Audience

Positive transference can be so subtle and pervasive that we can take advantage of it without realizing it. In this case, clients fall into an illusion that we are wiser and somehow better than they are, and we can fall right in there with them. We may act in a way that we wouldn't if we met the same person at a party. It can be appealing to have an attentive audience that defers to us. In the client's presence, we may imagine that we're so wise, we have such interesting stories to tell, our opinions and thoughts on just about anything are especially meaningful. When we allow that to happen, we have forgotten that the client is the star of the show, not us. (And as will be discussed later in the chapter, when we respond to clients' deference toward us as if we were entitled, we are in countertransference.)

Clients may put up with the practitioner's self-centeredness the same way, perhaps, that they put up with their parents'. It's survival. Would anyone risk offending someone who holds the key to helping or hindering them? Clients come to us seeking relief for pain or imbalance; sometimes they are desperate. Who would risk offending their bodyworker?

When we mistake positive transference for reality, when we buy into the illusion that we are better than the client, we lose our curiosity about the client—and we lose our effectiveness. What are the client's strengths and dreams? What pain is he ready to release? What does he want from the session? Clients know more about themselves than we do—sometimes they simply don't know that they know. Our job is to help them find the best in themselves, not to impose our own needs and egos.

Our curiosity and compassion go out the window when we pretend to be all-knowing or when we forget that the session belongs to the client. Even if a client needs to put us on a pedestal, we have to find ways to let them know that, while we are competent, we are merely consultants who have certain gifts. We don't possess God-like knowledge. At best, we know a small amount about a small area of the human condition.

Signs of Transference: Lost Souls

Don't we have some clients who really do like us, clients we have a great connection with—and isn't that OK? That's a good question. Are our sessions with them about us or about them? Are they lost souls coming to hear what a guru has to say or are we the ones who listen with curiosity and interest to what they bring to a session?

There are clients who try hard to please us, and that can feel good. But by basking in the glow of our own egos, we can miss the desperation underneath their efforts to please. Certified Feldenkrais trainer Paul Rubin, talks about clients who are at a time in their lives when they feel like "lost souls":

> Many people are at a choice point of "Do I
> find myself, or do I find someone I can see as

more powerful with whom I can have a dependent relationship?" It's always up to us to guide people back to finding their independence.

It's natural and therapeutic for clients to be dependent and look up to us at certain times. Also, most of us have had times in our lives when we felt like lost souls. However, if our practices are full of people who call us after hours, people who constantly lean on us, then we need to take a look at what's going on. Are we getting our own emotional needs met by cultivating dependency in clients? It's not our job to run our clients' lives. As a colleague, Janet Zimmerman, so aptly put it, "We have to remember that we're just the hired hands."

Signs of Transference: Sexual Feelings

Crushes are a common form of transference and it's easy to think that they are about us. They really aren't. Crushes don't mean that clients want romantic relationships with their practitioners. Rather, the client's unconscious is using the practitioner (in an appropriate, therapeutic way) to deal with deep issues. Clients may be working out personal issues about intimacy, about sexuality or about relationships. They may see in us the hidden parts of themselves—such as their own strength or their own compassion. Our work with such clients, perhaps our acceptance of them has awakened something, but their feelings aren't really about us.

Marion Rosen, founder of Rosen Method bodywork, uses the term "stand in" to describe what we are to our clients:

> I am 84 years old and when a 30-year-old male client tells me he is in love with me, I tell him

that this feeling has arisen in him from the work we are doing together and that I am just a "stand in" to enable him to do the inner work he needs to do.

If the client with a crush is an age and gender that we are usually attracted to, the situation can be more dangerous; it may make it easier both to misinterpret the intentions and to return the interest. If we are drawn to doing that, we need to seek outside help to sort it out. It's unethical to take advantage of a client's romantic transference feelings for us.

Negative Transference: What Did *I* Do?

With negative transference, we sometimes have the feeling of, "But I didn't do anything." Or, "Why does that bother her? It doesn't bother anyone else."

Imagine an adult client, who, as a child was beaten by a parent. Now he (and of course, the client could be a "she") is undressed or half-dressed and lying in a vulnerable position. The practitioner is looming over him about to do something unfamiliar and strange to his body. Just as his father was supposed to take care of him, so this bodyworker is supposed to be helping. On some level, usually not conscious, the client may be afraid of being hurt or overpowered again. Such a client may express anxiety by being unusually sensitive to touch or pulling away at the slightest pain. He may ask nervous questions about what we are doing or what our credentials are. Or he may go numb and be unresponsive to the work. As practitioners, such anxiety or lack of response may irritate us or confuse us, but if we understand transference, we can realize that the client is simply afraid of being hurt again.

Not every client who is wary or overly sensitive has physical (or sexual) abuse in his background. We may never know a client's reason for mistrusting us. But we make a mistake when we react to his anxiety with impatience, defensiveness or judgment.

Although negativity from the client may seem to be an attack or threat, it usually isn't any more about us than positive transference is. Human nature being what it is, we often see negative transference (the client is critical of us or doesn't trust us) as the client's problem, as some kind of character defect, while seeing positive transference (the client thinks we're wonderful) as a natural response to our winning personality. Neither perception is quite accurate. And neither perception is without a grain of truth.

Sometimes It *Is* About You

Knowing the dynamics of transference doesn't give us license to dismiss clients' complaints or criticisms as simply their old unresolved issues. If we keep getting the same kinds of negative feedback, it probably *is* about us. Understanding transference should make us more respectful of and sensitive to clients, not less.

There's truth in both positive and negative transference, but that truth is usually about our professional selves, not our private selves. Clients who love us may be responding to the fact that, during our hourly session, we are caring, concerned and sensitive to their needs. However, if clients knew us in our personal lives, they would have a fuller, more human and less idealized picture of us. By the same token, the client who has trouble trusting us may be responding to problems with our professional persona. For instance, they may be reacting to our carelessness about professional conduct—such as always being late. If punctuality is important to them, clients could focus on our lateness and overlook other ways that we are careful and professional. They could form a biased picture of us as a person who is generally inconsiderate and uncaring.

Dealing with Transference

If we don't know how to work with "difficult" clients, we can make the transference worse. And if we don't know how to work with adoring clients, we can get into trouble too. At the least, we miss an opportunity to help them achieve another stage of awareness. If we decline to take on their adoration, we may help them see that their feelings say more about them than they do about us.

The first rule is—and this is one of the rare times the word "rule" is used in this book—don't talk to clients about what we imagine their transference to be. We don't want to say, "You're just upset with me because you're still mad at your mother," or, "You have a crush on me because you need a strong father figure."

First, we don't really know what's causing their behavior. Next, we have to remember that transference is unconscious: the client may not know what we're talking about and may find it confusing or annoying. It's patronizing to tell clients our notions about their motivations. It assumes both that we know more about them than they do and that we have a license to talk about psychological dynamics with them. A client coming to us for a relaxing massage, a balancing structural integration session or an enlivening hour of movement work probably doesn't have an interest in our psychological theories.

Our job, as manual therapists faced with a strong negative or positive transference, is to be extra crisp about boundaries and to pay close attention to the framework* (framework is the nuts and bolts of a session—being on time, being consistent about fees and scheduling; framework is discussed at length in Chapter Four). If the client is already in "transference" love with us, we don't want to change the relationship and make it social. We don't want to accept her invitation to a party. If the client is already uncomfortable with us, tighter boundaries and care with the therapeutic environment can help her feel safer. The more we keep boundaries clear, the less chance of transference becoming destructive to the therapeutic relationship.

By our behavior, we can let clients know that this is a therapeutic situation—that we aren't an abusive parent *or* a savior and that the power is in their hands. Sometimes we want to tell them that more directly. We can use phrases like, "I'm just a consultant. You're the expert on your own body."

Be respectful of crushes and be respectful of the fears and complaints of a "difficult" client. We don't know where any of these feelings originate in clients. We don't know what their histories are or what deep aspects have been stirred. A colleague tells this story:

> A client complained about being poked by my fingernails, and I debated a minute before deciding to do anything about them. I'd just gotten a manicure—lovely red nails—and I'd just seen my favorite teacher, who also had long

---

*For definition, see page 228.

nails, work without pain to her client. Nevertheless, I decided to file my nails and was glad I did. Later in the session, my client told me that when she was a child, her mother would punish her by actually cutting her skin with her long red fingernails.

There's nothing mysterious about transference. Even in our daily lives, we imagine things about people we don't really know and have expectations about how people will act that are based on our past experiences with others. In a situation that has a built-in power difference, the transference can be more intense. The way we handle it can either help the client resolve old issues or make things worse. And how well we handle it can depend on our awareness of our own psychological history.

Countertransference

In this last section, I've started talking about countertransference without naming it. Countertransference is when we allow our own unresolved issues, feelings and needs to intrude into a session; we unconsciously transfer onto the client unresolved feelings and attitudes from *our* past relationships. It's when we act on a client's crush, rather than realizing that the client doesn't really want an intimate relationship with us. It's also when we respond to a client's criticism with annoyance and defensiveness, rather than professional objectivity.

Transference, if not seen for what it is, easily leads to countertransference; that is, the client may respond to us based on unconscious attitudes and feelings, and we may then respond back based on our unconscious feelings and attitudes.

Here's an example:

> Both client and practitioner are perfectionists—both feel that they never measured up to their parents' expectations and both still carry that insecurity. The practitioner, meaning to give information and sympathy, says to the client, "Boy, you're tight in your upper back." The client hears it as a parental criticism of his ability to take care of himself and responds with an irritated, "That's what you're supposed to help me with!" The practitioner hears that as a criticism of her professional skills and mumbles an exasperated, "I'm doing the best I can."
>
> An example of a more therapeutic response from the practitioner might be to say cheerfully, "You're right—it is what I'm supposed to do! I was merely wanting to let you know that it looks like you've been under a good deal of stress."

What we can reasonably expect from clients is some form of payment and that they treat us with respect. As long as they aren't abusively insulting or disrespectful, clients should be free to complain, become enamored of us, improve, not improve and generally go at their own pace without our taking it personally. If we expect certain kinds of validation—that they get better at a certain rate so we can feel like "good" practitioners, that they praise our work each session—that is countertransference and not useful. If we're constantly disappointed and angry with "resistive" clients, that's a red flag that signals that we have issues that we need to talk out with a more experienced professional.

The intimacy of bodywork triggers deep emotions and old feelings, and we are as much a part of that unconscious soup as the client. We can lose our objectivity in a second. Any strong feelings about a client—anger, chronic annoyance or even love—can signal that we are lost in countertransference. Another common red flag for countertransference is feeling tired or drained when we work with certain clients. We need to be curious about any negative reactions to clients and get help with understanding them.

What about loving our clients? Isn't it natural that we open our hearts to our clients? One way to distinguish healthy from unhealthy affection for clients is the extent to which they have become "special" to us. Do we give extra attention to what we're wearing if we are seeing them that day? Do we make exceptions for them that we don't for other clients? Do we give them extra time, rearrange our schedule to accommodate them, or let their bills slide? Do we go out of our way to help them with an outside problem? In other words, do we bend our own boundaries for this client?

A colleague relates:

> I was attracted to one of my new clients and at first, wasn't conscious of it. After a few sessions, I began to have signs of countertransference: I always looked forward to her session with some excitement and felt "high" at the end. I made a point of telling her about upcoming events that might be of interest to her and realized that this was in hopes that I might "accidentally"

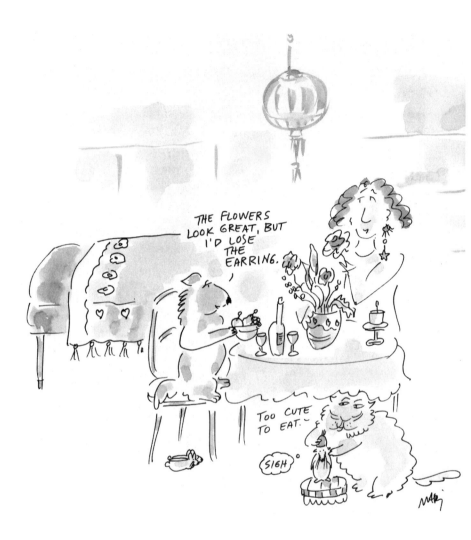

LOOKING FORWARD TO A CLIENT'S SESSION WITH EXCITEMENT IS A RED FLAG FOR COUNTER TRANSFERENCE ISSUES.

bump into her. She had a busy work life and I often came in earlier than I usually do to accommodate her. After I became aware of what I was doing, I discussed the attraction with my supervisor and was able to regain my balance with this client.

If we imagine that we are the only one who can truly understand a particular client, or that we are the only one who can help this client, we are in trouble. If we see ourselves as "rescuing" a helpless client, that's a red flag too.

As for negative countertransference, aren't some people just annoying? Perhaps. But it also could be that another practitioner would find them endearing or it could be that our "annoying client" is simply anxious and responding to our careless framework. Do we think a particular client has come to irritate us and make the day seem longer? Or do we sense that she is needing more from us and doesn't know what it is or how to ask for it?

Clients we see as difficult or demanding are often trying to mask their underlying fear, neediness or confusion. Because of that, the therapeutic response to these clients is actually just the opposite of our natural inclination. Most of us would be naturally inclined to be impatient and have a get-over-it attitude with such a client. However, to really settle this client down, we need to respond with attentiveness and concern, to ask for extra feedback about whether she is comfortable—how's the room temperature, does she want a deeper or lighter pressure, what else does she need to help her relax? It's easy to be caring with an appreciative client; picky clients are the true test of our compassion.

Dealing with Countertransference

Countertransference happens constantly. It's not a question of "if," but rather it's a question of when and how, and what kind of people we most easily over-react to. And once we think we've got our inner responses to clients figured out, someone walks through the door who turns us upside down, who makes us wonder why we feel mad, fascinated or exhausted. Working with our own transference (countertransference) is an ongoing learning process.

One of the best ways to learn to recognize when we are hooked by a client is to get professional supervision. Probably 90 percent of supervision's benefits are to help us untangle our countertransference and deal with our feelings related to our clients' transference. (See Chapter Ten for a discussion of supervision.)

> A practitioner found herself unusually annoyed with a client—a woman who was slightly older than the practitioner and who seemed sweet but passive. After talking with her supervisor, the practitioner realized that her feelings were related to her anger over her mother's passivity. She was able to work with her client more objectively once she realized the reason for her dislike and how inappropriate it was.

Talking over our responses to clients with a supervisor can help us gain the objectivity we need to be skilled in our client relationships. A supervisor can help us know, for instance, when and how to refer a client to someone else. (Getting supervision from a trained professional is not psychotherapy; supervisors help us understand our dynamics as they relate to our professional selves.) If we've done our best to find compassion for a client but are still constantly irritated, we're not helping such a client by continuing to work with him. Likewise, if we've discussed our feelings of attraction to a client and those feelings are still intruding into a session, we need to refer that client to another practitioner.

Paying attention to framework and boundaries provides safety for us as practitioners dealing with countertransference. We are human and always have unresolved issues, old wounds and insecurities. That's the reason we have professional boundaries and framework—so that when we wander off course, we can notice it and be curious about it : "Wonder why I'm willing to come in at 7 a.m. for this client when I don't usually work before 9 a.m." It could be a valid reason or it could be something else. Are we responding to a real need, or are we too intimidated to ask the client to fit into our schedule? Or are we emotionally seduced by him? When we find areas where we've strayed from our usual boundaries and framework, we can then correct our course.

Practitioners who regularly consult with a professional clinician* find that it helps them sort out these issues and makes their jobs easier. Strong positive or negative feelings about a client are red flags. Good supervision can help turn those annoyances or infatuations into solid learning experiences.

Hearts and Minds

The giving and receiving of bodywork can touch our hearts and cloud our minds. For both us and our clients, bodywork brings up unconscious material that can interfere with the

---

*For definition, see page 227.

therapeutic relationship. Clients get mad at us, clients fall in love with us, we get mad or love them back. Our role is to sort out those feelings in a way that empowers clients and helps them heal old wounds. Our job is to do our best to keep our own issues from intruding into the therapeutic process.

Clear boundaries and a sturdy framework help both parties handle their transference and countertransference. They orient us and bring clarity to the murkiness that arises from unresolved personal history. When we strive to be consistent and even-handed, we can identify our red flags more quickly and get help when heading down the wrong path. It takes careful thought, training and determination not to take advantage of the power inherent in the therapeutic relationship.

Framework: Nuts and Bolts

Chapter Four

Framework issues can sound dry and dull. Who wants to talk about the joy of starting sessions on time and the delights of clean sheets? "Framework" refers to the small ways we define our practices as professional—time boundaries, fees, the appearance of the therapy room, confidentiality, etc. Framework is more important and deserves more thought than most of us realize. Many a manual therapy career has suffered because of carelessness about the details that make clients comfortable.

Our clients are vulnerable and need good boundaries in order to trust us. Framework details are the nuts and bolts of good boundaries. Clients care about those issues more than we may be aware:

> I asked my old friend Robbie what made her a loyal client of her massage therapist. "She's very competent," she said. Since Robbie is an art history professor and doesn't know effleurage from petrissage, I was curious how she came to that conclusion. She thought for a minute and said, "Her tapes are long enough."
>
> She meant that the massage therapist was careful to time her music to last for the whole session, so that she didn't have to fumble around with the music and interrupt the flow. She

added that the room is always clean and tidy, the table is heated and the therapist doesn't talk unless Robbie initiates it. Also, she never gives a massage-by-the-numbers, but always homes in on where my friend's aches and pains are that week.

Our clients know little about the technical part of our work. Our offices are foreign territory, and the only way they can judge our competence and caring is by our professional behavior and whether they feel safe with us.

The ability to create an atmosphere within which the client can make use of our work is crucial. We may rush to learn the latest techniques and pride ourselves on our sensitivity, but our effectiveness can depend on whether or not, in a manner of speaking, our tapes are long enough.

Holding the Space

Some practitioners call it "holding the space;" others, "creating a container." They recognize that clients need to have a special environment that's focused solely on their well-being. More than simply putting out some crystals and playing soft music, we need to take care of all the details that make us professional. We need, for example, to start and end on time, to be consistent about what we charge and to keep our attention on our clients. Careless framework can interfere with the therapeutic process. A colleague reports:

> I used to be a massage therapist in a holistic center in which no one had an assigned office. Instead, you used whatever room was available at the time. Sometimes my client and I

had to wait ten or fifteen minutes until a room was available. We rarely worked in the same room two times in a row. The other practitioners and I often talked about how uptight our clients seemed to be, how long it took them to relax. Now I see that their difficulty letting go was probably a response to our erratic set-up. How could they relax in such an unstable environment?

Sometimes clients aren't even conscious of what is making them uncomfortable. They just feel out of kilter. Change can make clients uncomfortable without knowing why. When we have to see clients at a time other than their usual one, we may notice that they then behave differently—pickier, more off balance, more insecure in some way. We may have to make an extra effort to help them feel comfortable, or we may need to make a comment to show them that we know how unsettling even such a small adjustment can be. Most reassuring of all, we can make sure things are back to normal by the next session.

Framework Basics

The following pages present framework guidelines. If they sound too much like rules, realize that they really are acts of kindness toward a vulnerable client. They are also small acts of self-discipline that will make our work lives run more smoothly. Often, clients react to careless framework by acting nervous, fussy or simply not coming back. Practitioners react by feeling harried and drained by the end of the day. Those of us who are not already honoring these guidelines may want to try them out and see if we don't notice a positive difference. (Practitioners who have been pretty scattershot about framework for a long time will need to be consistently careful for some time before noticing a difference.)

There *are* good practitioners who routinely violate one or more of these precepts, yet seem to have healthy practices. These people usually get by on superb technical skills or charisma—clients will sometimes forgive our other omissions if we have the balance of a great personality or we're good "fixers." Yet even in those cases, clients will notice and respond positively if those practitioners start attending to framework issues. And the practitioners will find they have fewer "difficult" clients and more energy at the end of the day.

> An excellent and popular massage therapist worked for years out of a room in her home that was less than neat—it was a cluttered mess. Order did not reign in that office. In spite of that, she was popular because she was a good listener and a sensitive bodyworker, plus she was professional in every other way.
>
> A few months ago, she complained that her work seemed to take more and more energy over the years. I suggested that she try simply tidying up the room. I thought that she wouldn't have to work as hard to create a professional atmosphere if the room said it for her. It was a small change, but she reported that cleaning the room made a difference. She looks forward to her work more in this neater, more professional office and reports that new clients seem to settle in and relax faster.

Some practitioners have great personalities and/or amazing skills. For the rest of us, the majority, who are charismatically-impaired and less-than-dazzling technicians, attention to framework will balance our shortcomings. Consistency, reliability and care for the client can go a long way toward a good solid, satisfying practice. And we'll last longer in this profession. The guidelines* that follow are some nuts and bolts of good framework.

Sessions start and end on time.

Time boundaries help make a safe "container"—they are part of what defines the experience as other than social and puts safe limits on the therapeutic relationship. Starting on time is respectful of both our time and the client's.

Picture this: You're the client and you've been looking forward to your massage (or shiatsu session, Reiki treatment, or whatever) all day. You've arranged your day to be there on time at 3 p.m.—you're tired, you're sore, your back hurts. You arrive and your practitioner is on the phone. The last client's dirty sheets are still on the table. Or you arrive and the practitioner greets you at the door and shows you to a warmly welcoming room that is ready to go. How do those two scenarios compare in feeling?

Ending on time is just as important. "If you don't end your session on time, your client will never trust you," says Sandra Wooten, director of Rosen Method Center Southwest. Clients like to know what to expect. Unpredictable practitioners make clients uneasy. If we go long one session because the client is in pain, she may think we'll go short next time if she's not.

---

*Nan Narboe, L.C.S.W, "Working with What You Can't Get Your Hands On," (Portland, Ore., 1985)

Even if clients are still experiencing intense emotion or pain, ending at the agreed-on time provides comforting structure. Lengthening sessions because there is still pain or emotion tells clients that they need to be "rescued" and that we don't trust either them or the process. It can tell them that their pain is as overwhelming to us as it is to them.

Being consistent about time has many advantages. It makes it easier for us to gauge when we are caught in countertransference, for instance. If we're usually consistent, but find ourselves always wanting to go over or under the usual amount of time with a certain client, that can tell us we need to look at why we are treating that client differently. It also makes it easier to monitor ourselves in other ways. If we want to take extra time with *every* client, we may be trying too hard, and if we want to cut the session short with every client, we may be approaching burn-out.

What "ending on time" means varies from practitioner to practitioner. Those who are doing emotionally-oriented bodywork, such as Rosen Method or Rubenfeld Synergy, are careful to end at the hour. Many manual therapists don't schedule precisely on the hour or hour and a half; they have some leeway for how long it will take to get their work done or the client's relative speed in getting dressed and undressed. Most practitioners that I interviewed thought that fifteen minutes was enough leeway. It's also a good idea, even if our practices aren't full, to schedule as if they are. It's good discipline and it shows the client that we value our time.

Being consistent about time doesn't mean that we need to be rigid about time; sometimes a client is in an unusual crisis. A massage therapist told of taking an extra thirty minutes with a client whose mother just died. (The therapist wasn't disrupting other clients' schedules by doing so.) A bodyworker said she took extra time with a client who had come from another state. If we are late to a session, we want to make up that time to the client—either that day or at a later time. But exceptions should be rare and thought-out. Our practices run much more smoothly, and our clients are more secure when we start and end on time.

Sessions occur at the same time and place at regular intervals.

Although we're not in control of whether our clients come back regularly, we can be aware of the importance of consistency and try to keep them in the same time slot. If we have to bounce a client out of a regular time or if we're relocating our practice to a different office, we want to be aware of keeping the other parts of the framework on an even keel. Moves and changes can upset clients without their fully realizing it. It's enough for a client to have his body changing without having the environment whirling around too. The more stability we can build into the framework, the better.

Nothing interrupts a session.

All of these guidelines are based on the central idea that being professional means that the focus is on our clients. They are paying for our time and attention. There's rarely a good reason to answer the phone during a session. Perhaps if we knew that the Nobel Peace Prize committee was going to call during that hour... but even so, we would need to warn the client of a possible interruption.

A practitioner who works at home needs to keep the environment as free of interruptions as possible—for example, put a

73

"Do Not Disturb" sign on the front door and advise friends not to drop by. If an interruption is unavoidable (the sink is stopped up and the plumber is coming), we can let clients know before the session starts that there may be a brief interruption of the session and let them know that we will make up the time lost. If we know ahead of time that the session may be interrupted, it's best to call clients and forewarn them before their session.

Practitioners should do their utmost to see that no one walks in on a session. Clients will be jarred by that, no matter who the intruder is. A friend relates:

> One of my most uncomfortable massages was from a woman who worked out of her living room and had a three-year-old child. Throughout the massage, whenever I opened my eyes, I'd see the curious little girl peeking in. She didn't say anything or actively take her mother's attention, but just knowing that she was looking at me took away my privacy.

Nothing is said outside of the session

Nothing that goes on in our sessions, neither what clients say nor their physical reactions, is carried outside. We don't discuss it outside the session with the client (boundaries), and we don't tell other people about it (confidentiality).

When we see clients in another setting, we may be tempted to talk about the work we're doing together: "Are you still sore?" "I hope you're feeling better." Those may seem like innocent remarks, but when we carry our therapeutic role to another setting, we confuse the boundaries. For instance, when clients are having a session, they're relaxed and in an altered state. We violate their privacy when we bring information from that situation into another setting.

If we see clients (past or present) in an outside setting, standard protocol is to not approach them. If they approach us, then we can acknowledge them and be as friendly as we normally would. If we know we're going to run into clients outside, we can let them know that we will let them initiate contact.

Those of us who don't do emotionally-oriented work or transformational work* sometimes work with friends or acquaintances. To help keep the boundaries clear, we can let them know that what goes on in the session needs to stay there and that if they have questions about the work, they can set up a separate time to talk about it rather than using social time.

The Internet has opened up new areas for boundary complications. Some Internet servers have features that enable customers to know when another customer is online and then "chat" with him. Internet boundaries should follow the same guidelines as in-person boundaries, even though there's a kind of anonymity about socializing online. We still want to avoid having anything but polite social conversation with clients when we accidentally bump into them outside the office, even if the connection is electronic. We might want to be careful about making our personal screen names available to clients.

Violations of confidentiality can seem innocent. Mary and Susie are friends and both are clients of Joe, the massage therapist. Mary says to Joe, "I haven't seen Susie in a while. How's she doing?" It's easy for Joe to say, "Oh, she's still having a hard

---

*For definition, see page 230.

time with her marriage." But if he does, he's broken confidentiality with Susie and to make it worse, now Mary knows that he passes on clients' private information to other people. Even "Susie's feeling great" is a violation. To keep clear framework, Joe can say lightly, "Oh, you know I can't talk about my other clients." Clients who are friends with other clients will sometimes test us—usually not consciously—to see if we will talk about their friend to them (and therefore, talk to the friend about them).

Confidentiality will be discussed further in Chapter Five.

Clients are unaware of each other.
Therapists who do classic psychotherapy or psychoanalysis arrange their schedules and office entrances and exits so that clients don't see each other. One client leaves from one door at ten minutes to the hour and the next one comes in a different door on the hour. The idea is to maintain clients' privacy and cut down on the potential for their positive or negative imaginings about the therapist's relationship with other clients.

> Waiting to get a session from a much-loved teacher, I saw him walk out of his previous session with his arm around his client, chatting in a friendly way. Great annoyance and dismay arose in me and I realized I was spinning off into an internal dialogue of: "He doesn't do that with me. He likes that other client better than he likes me. He probably doesn't like me at all."

Because I had a solid history of trusting that teacher, the

situation didn't interfere with my session, but it could have been disruptive. It could have been one of those sessions when the practitioner didn't know why the client was being "resistive."

Most of us weren't taught to schedule our clients so that they arrive and leave without seeing each other, but it's a good idea. We don't know how it will affect one client to see us giving a hug to the previous client at the door: it may mean nothing, but it may be confusing and upsetting. Arranging for clients to leave without bumping into someone else is also considerate of the fact that, as they leave our offices, they're not always in a frame of mind to deal with other people. They may be tearful or think their hair looks messy, or they may still be in an altered state and not wanting to cope with polite chit-chat.

The key idea here is that clients don't need to be aware of our professional relationships with other clients. For this reason, we don't name our clients to each other and when we are with one client, we don't want to even mention the existence of other clients. We want to create a setting in which each client can feel that he or she is the total focus of our attention. There's probably not a client in the world who is interested in seeing us warmly embrace another client or hearing us talk about another client. Why run the risk of stirring up something that will interfere with the client's process?

Practitioners don't ask clients to attend to their needs.
It's never appropriate to ask clients to attend to our needs. We might be tempted to do this in an obvious way, such as trying to get sympathy about our difficult divorce, or asking for advice about their areas of expertise. I talk about the obvious variety in the first chapter. Practitioners with good intentions

77

can be misled by the notion that it's helpful to clients to be open with them about our personal issues. Actually, it can be a distraction in what is *their* time. What is really helpful to clients is giving them our full attention, and not dragging our personal lives into the session, or asking people who are paying us to also give us emotional support or free advice.

There may be times when sharing something from our personal lives is useful. The decision about whether to do this must be based on what will be helpful to the client. For instance, a client that we've known for a long time may feel shut out or insulted if we never give out any personal information.

There are other, less obvious ways we ask clients to take care of our needs. We might say things like, "Boy, I've had a rough day," "I can't stand this hot weather," or "I'm so tired from last night." Even these subtle messages can create problems. Maybe we've had a hard day, but so have they—they've come to us so that we can help their day be easier. When they hear something that sounds like we're not up to snuff that day, it can interfere with their ability to trust us and let go.

Clients are paying us to put aside our personal needs and do what's best for them. Personal revelations from the practitioner can be off-putting. They may begin to see us, in small ways, as needy and inadequate to handle their problems.

We're not being deceptive when we keep our personal needs out of the session: it's just good professional manners. We are not arrogantly pretending that we don't have needs, we are simply being appropriate to the professional setting.

When is Framework Important?

Framework is always important, with all clients. The following are some reasons why it's important with specific groups:

New clients: The first appointment is crucial for setting a professional tone. Clients put off by sloppy framework in the first session just don't come back. No second chances. Lateness with a regular client can be dismissed as a momentary lapse, but with a brand-new client, it can imply indifference or incompetence.

Regular clients: Regular clients get used to their routines and their one hour a week feels like a safe haven. So we try to avoid taking clients out of their pattern. If we have to change the framework—move offices or raise fees, for example—we may even lose clients if we're not sensitive in presenting those changes. We need to give clients ample notice (a month or so) about major changes.

Clients undergoing transformational processes—structural and/or emotional: In deeply transformational bodywork, when clients' physical (and emotional) patterns are shifting, they need a stable therapeutic environment. The more we expect to access deep emotional material, the more care we need to take with framework. It's not merely a personal whim that makes Rosen Method teacher, Karen Anderson, spend extra time before a session making sure that sheets are neat and evenly balanced on the table. An ordered environment helps clients allow their feelings to emerge.

Mentally disturbed clients: If we're working with clients whose internal process is chaotic, we need to be more attentive to external boundaries. This can be difficult because their own sense of boundaries is usually so scattered that they tend not to honor ours. They may want special exceptions:

> A colleague working with a woman who suffered from a borderline personality disorder found that the client wanted her to (1) lower her fee, (2) give her a ride to the session, (3) work only with one specific area, even though my friend's methods called for a whole body approach, and (4) let her cancel sessions on the day of the session.

Gentle firmness and consistency are settling for these clients. The more we make exceptions, the more we're asking for trouble.

Clients who have been traumatized or who are in physical distress: Fear and pain make us more sensitive to orderliness and kindness in the environment. Clients with post traumatic stress disorder are vigilant and watchful, expecting danger behind every door. Clients frightened by chronic physical pain are like wounded animals who have retreated into a corner. Both kinds of clients are hypersensitive to any perceived imbalance in the therapeutic relationship. Small framework errors or lapses in attention can seem to them to be confusion or indifference.

People with whom we have another relationship: We can be tempted to be careless about framework with people we know: "I don't have to have the room ready—it's only my buddy Bob." We actually need to be *more* crisp with our boundaries in such cases to help friends with the confusion of switching roles. (See Chapter Nine on Dual Relationships.)

People who've been sexually abused: Extra attention to framework is necessary for clients who have been sexually abused. At the same time, because their own boundaries may be confused, they may push the edges—being flirtatious with us or asking for special treatment.

Those categories cover just about everyone. Framework is important for all clients, for one reason or another.

Bending Framework, A Red Flag

When we bend our professional boundaries, we encourage others to treat us as if we're not professionals. When our boundaries become Swiss cheese, we make holes that clients can fall through.

Les Kertay, clinical psychologist and chair of the Rolf Institute's ethics committee, says that making special exceptions for clients is always a red flag for the practitioner. One of the main ways people get into big trouble with clients (ethics complaints, for instance) or even small trouble (the client doesn't come back or becomes a "difficult" client) is through treating the client as "special" in some way.

> The only time in my twenty years of practice when I didn't get paid was by a client for whom I had made exception after exception. I allowed my judgment to be clouded because (1) she had a large and challenging area of scar tissue on her chest and neck from a traumatic childhood injury, (2) she was a struggling single mother, (3) she said she was in a great deal of pain.

Rushing in to rescue her, I discounted my fee substantially and would see her at times when I didn't usually schedule sessions. She never seemed to get relief from the pain, and that would double my desire to fix her. The last time I saw her, I agreed to work on my birthday although I had planned to take the day off. To make it worse, I was giving her a discount. At the end of the session, she said she didn't have any checks with her and that she would mail me the fifty dollars. That was the last I heard from her.

Stiffed on my birthday—it's a lesson I remember. I had created a framework disaster.

Would it have been hard-hearted not to make an exception for a client in great pain? We want to distinguish between the client who is sincerely in a crisis and the client who has a pattern of being manipulative. That can be a difficult judgment call, but often there are clues. For example, there are clients who call and say that they are in terrible distress and must be seen right away. But if the practitioner says, for instance, "I can't see you Sunday, but I have an opening at 10 a.m. on Monday," they will invariably say something like, "Oh, I can't then. That's when I get my hair cut," or take the dog to the vet, etc. Or there are clients who describe awful pain and want to be seen immediately. When the practitioner asks how long they've had the pain, they'll say, "six months." This doesn't mean that their pain isn't real—but it may mean that we don't need to rearrange our schedules to see them right away.

We don't do clients a favor when we let them hook us into ignoring our own framework policies. We also don't need to judge clients who want to be treated in a special way. The client who didn't pay me was just dealing with a difficult situation in an unhealthy way that she'd learned a long time ago. It was a mistake for me to continue to treat her in a special way and it wasn't helpful to her. No wonder she never seemed to benefit from the work. People heal best when they have a safe container, and I didn't provide that for her. She never knew where my boundaries were.

If someone has been injured or is in emotional crisis, depending on the circumstances and our schedule, we may want to make an exception for him. Special exceptions need to be carefully considered and consistent. Experienced practitioners will develop their own guidelines about what circumstances will warrant bending the standard framework, and they will then avoid going outside their own rules. Firm framework saves energy and stress and provides comfort for both practitioner and client.

Framework from the Beginning: Setting the Stage

Our work with clients begins long before they walk through the door. It starts with the first phone call or even the first time they see our business card. We need to take care how we present ourselves from the very beginning.

Business Cards

Business cards usually won't make or break a practice. I've seen unimpressive cards for practitioners with prosperous practices.

However, cards are one more piece of information about us and if prospective clients see them (for example, on the bulletin board at the health food store), we want them to have a favorable impression and a clear understanding of our work.

Having a business card says that we're serious about our work. Also, the process of designing a card is often useful in that we have to figure out what tone we want to set and what we want people to know about us.

Our cards should clearly say what we do, without exaggeration. Some cards look like a smorgasbord: "Mary Smith— Hypnotherapy, Past life regression, Acupressure, Sports massage and Palm reading." That can be confusing to prospective clients, and they could also be skeptical that, unless Mary Smith is 103 years old, she can't be really good at all of those things.

Reaching Us

Unlike doctors, very few manual therapists have an office with a receptionist. Most of us have various combinations of beepers, voice mails and answering machines. The key is that we sound professional and are easily accessible, since these are usually our first contacts with prospective clients.

Boundaries come into play here. We want people to be able to reach us, yet not be given a tour of our personal lives. It's best to have a separate line or voice mail for our business and to have an answering machine message that's professional and to the point. Practitioners using their home phone as their work phone may have to sacrifice the desire to showcase their children, leave witty messages or impart their philosophy of life. Also, is there anyone who really likes listening to another person's favorite music when trying to leave a message? Someone shopping for a manual therapist usually appreciates a short, relevant message for business.

If we take and return business calls from a private line, we want to make sure the television isn't blaring in the background, or the children needing attention. Practitioners who take calls at home can use a screening device, like caller ID, so they can choose when to answer. A boyfriend answering the phone when it's a business call sends out more information about the practitioner's life than the client needs. A small child answering the phone might be endearing and it might be annoying. Five minutes of "Is your mommy home?" doesn't put clients in the mood to make an appointment. They may wonder if the practitioner's family life will interfere with her professional life in other ways.

The First Phone Call

The therapeutic relationship starts with the first call. Rob Bauer, Rubenfeld Synergist, notes, "Transference and countertransference are already in process during the first phone call. Clients are imagining things, intuiting things about you—whether you're sensitive, or whether you're single, or how excited you are about your work."

We want to be informative and reassuring, but not sound as if we're reading from a set speech. (For brand-new practitioners, it's a good idea to find out from a more experienced colleague what the most common questions about your work are. You don't want to stumble around when prospective clients ask you the benefits of your work. Rehearse.) We want to show people that we're listening to them, that we hear what they're saying about what motivated them to call. Some of these points sound obvious, but it's surprising how many experienced manual therapists could use some polish in their phone talk.

For the practitioner, much can be learned about clients in the initial phone call. Do they have trouble with boundaries? Do they, for instance, want to share a great deal of personal information or get advice? We need to start setting boundaries in that first call—letting them know that some issues are best dealt with during their office visit. Be careful about letting people take up an unusual amount of time on the phone; it sets a bad precedent.

The first phone call is an important opportunity to educate the client. We need to be crisp. For example, we can let the client know what appointments we *do* have open, rather than all the reasons we *can't* see them on Thursday at 3 p.m. We also have an opportunity to set the stage for the session:

> Arnold Katz, a massage therapist in Boston, says that, even in the first phone call, after a client has made an appointment, he explains what will happen in the session very thoroughly, so there's no mystery. He takes clients through the session step-by-step from the minute they come in the door—that he will take a physical history, that he will then leave the room so that they can get undressed, that they will lie under a sheet and be draped at all times, and so forth. He lets them know from the beginning that if they are uncomfortable in any way at any time, he wants to know right away.

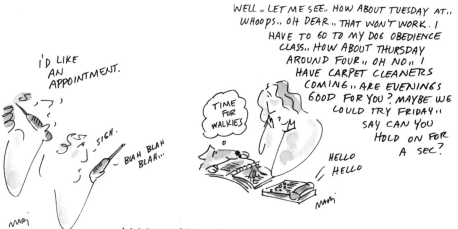

INSTEAD OF THIS...

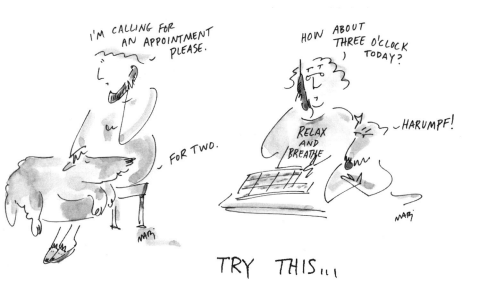

TRY THIS...

Home or Office?

Working out of an office, rather than a house, is more professional and feels safer to clients. A client reports:

> When I first started getting bodywork, I made
> an appointment with a male practitioner who
> had been well recommended. In spite of that,
> just knowing that he worked out of his house
> made me uncomfortable. When I went for that
> first appointment, I actually gave a friend the
> practitioner's address and said, "If I don't call
> you in two hours, call the police." The session
> went fine, but I want bodyworkers to know
> that their business can be affected if they work
> out of their homes.

Separating Work Space and Personal Life

The more we can separate our work and our personal lives, the better. If we work out of our homes, we want to use a room that's set aside just for our professional work. Again, the message needs to be that this is a space solely for the client.

There's no harm in having a couple of family pictures in the room—in fact, it can be reassuring to clients. However, some of the people I interviewed noted that practitioners need to be careful about making the room into a display of their personal spiritual beliefs. It can be a problem for clients. They may feel excluded if they don't share our beliefs or they may have judgments about our beliefs.

Getting the Room Ready

Clients love coming into a room that's all set up for them—

neat, warm sheets on the table and ready to go. Ready rooms are an immediate sign of our professionalism and caring.

One of the main things that makes clients uncomfortable is an unclean room or surroundings. Clients don't find it charming when the cat jumps on their bare back with sticky kitty-littered feet (true story). Or the room is obviously dirty. Or the bathroom is a mess. People these days are concerned about catching something. We want a balance between a room that smells antiseptic and a room that looks like germs may be lurking in every corner. We always want to be careful to wash our hands. If doctors forget to do it—and studies show that they do—my guess is that manual therapists do too.

Order and cleanliness in the environment aren't just a matter of being compulsive. After all, some people grow up with ideas about their bodies being "dirty" and may feel a heightened vulnerability when they get bodywork. People know that their bodies do embarrassing things—they sweat and make funny noises and are often out of conscious control. Clean, professional surroundings help clients to relax.

Framework At The End: Achieving Closure

We want to do our best to end our professional relationship with clients in a way that doesn't leave them with negative feelings that could color how they evaluate their entire time working with us.

Contacting Clients Who Quit

What do we do when a client suddenly stops coming to see us without letting us know why? Should we call the client? Should we write a note? There are so many variables here. Do we think the client was about to have a breakthrough and got scared? Do we think we may have offended the client in some way? There are conflicting ideas about how to handle this, ranging from, "Yes, you always want to let a client know that you're concerned," to "No, it's intrusive to contact a client who has stopped coming," to "It depends on the situation."

Here's an excellent example of a time to use a supervisor or a supervision group* to clarify our response to the situation. When someone stops seeing us abruptly, our decision about how to deal with it may be influenced by our personal feelings. We may, for instance, feel angry, rejected or just plain disappointed. Discussing our feelings with a supervisor can help us disentangle ourselves and decide how to handle the situation.

Moving Out of Town, Quitting Our Practices

If even small changes in our framework are disruptive to clients, what is it like for them when we leave town or quit our practices? If we terminate with clients carelessly, we leave them with a bad feeling about the whole experience of working with us or make them wary of going to another practitioner. For practitioners too, it's often emotionally difficult to leave. Getting supervision and support during this time can help make the transition smoother for the practitioner so that he/she can appropriately help clients weather the change.

Framework Matters

What individual clients need in order to feel safe will vary. There are guidelines, such as confidentiality, that are universally part of a professional code. Others may lend themselves to flexibility. For instance, in some cases, because of either the

---

*For definition, see page 229.

practitioner's personality or the client's, a cluttered treatment room may not make a difference. In other cases, messiness could make a client uncomfortable. The ultimate authority of framework is the client's experience. Does what we do make our clients tense or help them breathe easier?

Maintaining a stable framework will benefit us also. An inconsistent framework—variations in how long sessions run, special deals with fees, for instance—is energy-consuming for a practitioner.

While we want to be consistent and stable in our framework, experienced practitioners know total consistency is an ideal, rather than a reality. The point is not to become rigidly locked into rules, but to know that framework matters and to thoughtfully consider the ways we manage the nuts and bolts of our practice.

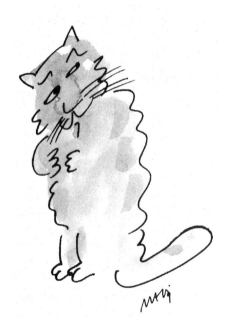

Ethics: From Theory to Practice

❈
Chapter Five

We often look at ethics in a simple way—what are the rules and how do we stay out of trouble? Although there are standards to guide us, ethical behavior can involve a delicate balancing act that has more to do with relationships and feelings than with black and white absolutes.

There are few hard-and-fast rules and we can follow them to the letter of the law and still get into some kind of trouble—offending a client or having a complaint lodged against us. The "right" thing to do can depend on the situation. We need to know and follow the standards of our state and national associations, but it's equally important to learn to make ethical decisions under any circumstance.

Making Ethical Decisions

Here are central questions we need to ask to determine whether an action is ethical:

- Does it keep the focus on the safety and well-being of the client?
- Is the practitioner being respectful of the power imbalance and/or the transference effect? Or using it to her/his own benefit?
- Does it create a dual relationship* and therefore, make the therapeutic relationship less clear?

---

*For definition, see page 228.

- Does it stay within the original contract with the client—are we exceeding either our area of expertise or the client's informed consent?
- Does it create a safer environment for the client or detract from it?
- Could this action lead to problems in the therapeutic relationship down the road?

Of these concerns, the first two are most important—keeping the focus on the client and not taking advantage of the transference.

Ethical Guidelines

Certain ethical rules and guidelines are standard parts of most associations' codes of ethics. With any guidelines, however, there are situations that require judgment calls on the part of the practitioner. Here are some examples of an ethical guideline and the judgment calls that could arise in following that guideline:

Sexual Relationships: The Ethical Standard

It's unethical to have a sexual relationship with a client. With an ex-client, it's unethical to use the affection, power or intimacy of the client/practitioner relationship to create a sexual relationship. It's also unethical to sexualize the relationship with a client by dressing seductively, flirting or making remarks that could be construed as sexual. (Sexual issues are complex and are discussed in more detail in Chapters Six and Seven.)

Sexual Relationships: Judgment Calls

At a party, you are talking with someone you have just met, someone you find attractive. The person learns that you are a bodyworker (or massage therapist or movement teacher) and wants to make an appointment. What do you do?

You have been working with a client for several months and you realize that you are starting to feel sexually attracted to him/her. What should you do?

We know that the absolute rule is not to date or have sexual relations with a client, but what about sexual attractions? It depends, for one thing, on how attracted we are:

- Is it just a passing thought?
- Is there a spark of sexual connection between you?
- Are you often aware of being sexually attracted to another person or is this a rare feeling—so that the attraction takes on greater meaning?
- Are you feeling emotionally off kilter, so that you might be more-than-usually tempted to act on an attraction?
- And if you are married or in a relationship, are you happy with the relationship?
- Do you know that you are capable of being attracted to a client without it interfering with your work?

We have to know ourselves and our limitations. The session should always focus on the client and not on our personal needs. If we have strong romantic/sexual feelings about a client, those feelings will usually intrude into the professional relationship. A strong attraction is a good issue to take to a supervisor for discussion.

We also need to consider the effect of transference. The decision to become someone's practitioner shouldn't be made casually. Once a person becomes a client (and often before they arrive on the table), transference begins, feelings are heightened on both sides. We have started to become, in their eyes (and perhaps in our own), a little larger than life—the compassionate care-giver, the heroic reliever of pain or the one to whom she can tell her painful secrets. Under those circumstances, clients are not as free to say "no." It's unethical to take advantage of the special feelings a client may have about us by trying to turn a professional relationship into a dating one.

Once someone becomes a client, we may never be able to have a normal social relationship with that person. If the work we do involves deep transformation or is psychologically-oriented, the possibilities for it being ethical to date ex-clients are slim. The effects of transference are simply too deep.

Even if we are "only" doing massage, once we become that person's practitioner, we have limited the relationship. Most associations' ethics require a wait of several months before a practitioner dates an ex-client. Regardless of the number of months that have passed, practitioners dating an ex-client would be a cause for concern and/or scrutiny in their professional circles. We're better off choosing whether this person will be part of our professional lives or part of our social lives.

In the first example, how do we decide whether to make the appointment? To start with, it's never a good idea to make an appointment or do business at a party. We can just offer the person our business card. That also gives us time to sort out our feelings and/or consult with a teacher or counselor trained in supervision. If we know we're not in danger of acting on our sexual attraction, we can take the person as a client, knowing that we are thereby eliminating the possibility of having a sexual relationship with him while he is a client. And we may be eliminating the possibility of ever ethically having a sexual relationship with him. If we're not sure whether we want to exclude that possibility, it's smart to buy time. For instance, when the person calls, we can simply say we don't have any appointments available. Given enough time, we can find our ethical bearings and decide whether to take that person as a client.

In the second situation, in which we become attracted to someone who is already a client, it's probably best to consult with a supervisor before making a decision. If we come to understand the reasons for the attraction, the feelings may dissipate. If they don't, then we may need to stop working with the client. Supervision is strongly suggested to help us with such situations. (Supervision is discussed in Chapter Ten.)

Prejudices: The Ethical Standard
We owe clients our care and attention. We may not connect with a person right away, but if we can't imagine ever having a caring attitude toward a particular client, we shouldn't work with him/her. If we have so many negative judgments or prejudices about a client that we could never have compassion for him, we cannot work with that client. We need to be on the alert for anything that interferes with our abilities to touch a client in a respectful, non-judgmental way. We are not just touching bodies—we're touching spirits.

Prejudices: Judgment Calls

> Your new client reveals that she/he belongs to
> a group that offends your belief system. (for
> instance, she/he is a gay rights advocate or a
> fundamentalist or a member of the N.R.A. or
> pro-choice.)
>
> Your new client does something you find very
> annoying. She/he talks constantly, never talks,
> has a whiny voice or talks very loudly.

We all constantly make positive and negative judgments about
people. We all have prejudices to some degree. The question is
how much such feelings interfere with our work. Sometimes
the judgments are minor and fleeting and dissipate as we get to
know the client. Sometimes they are so strong that we can't imagine ever having compassion or understanding for that client.

Not all of our clients are people with whom we would want to
be friends, but there should be something in us that connects
with something in them; they should touch our hearts. If that
connection is missing, we may not be the appropriate practitioner. Working with people we don't care for, or about whom
we have misgivings, can seriously compromise the safety of
the therapeutic environment. We may be inclined to be late,
to be less than present, to tune them out, to shortchange them
on time or to lack compassion.

We might know from the start that we can't work with a
client. We may have too strong a prejudice or too intense a
personal association, such as the client is gay and we are uncomfortable with homosexuality, or the client reminds us of

the handsome boyfriend who broke our hearts. If that is the case, we need to suggest that the client see someone else.

Or we may feel that we can work through the issue in a peer group* or with a supervisor. It's an excellent idea to have those already in place—to use peer groups and supervision as a preventive measure, and not wait until we're in trouble. If examining our attitudes in supervision doesn't change our negative feelings, then we need to refer the client to someone else or simply tell him we can't continue to work with him.

How to discontinue working with a client will be discussed later in this chapter. Nan Narboe, a psychotherapist who supervises manual therapy practitioners, suggests one way to make it easier:

> When you make the first appointment, tell your prospective client that the first few sessions will allow the client to decide whether she/he can effectively work with you and also allow you to decide whether your work is the most effective for this client. If you decide that you should not continue working with the client, you can then say, "I don't think my work will be as beneficial for you as X or Y" (other methods or other practitioners).

Every situation will be different. We can get professional help in deciding how best to discontinue our work with a client.

Taking Financial Advantage of a Client: The Ethical Standard
It's unethical to use the privilege of the client/practitioner relationship to profit financially. It's not ethical to exploit the

---

*For definition, see page 229.

relationship by using it to influence the client to buy a product or service or to make any investment from which the practitioner would profit.

Taking Financial Advantage of a Client: Judgment Calls
> Your friend is a distributor for a supplement that is high quality and said to boost energy and help certain physical problems. You have taken these vitamins and feel very enthusiastic about their value. Your friend thinks it would be a good idea for you to become a distributor and sell them to your clients.

Is it ethical to sell products to a client? Some professional bodywork associations ban their members from doing so. Others don't put restrictions on this practice. Some practitioners have no qualms about selling vitamins, blue-green algae or magnets to clients. Others don't think it's a good idea. How do we decide what is right?

Looking back at the questions that determine ethical actions at the first of the chapter, there are a number of potential problems with selling to clients. While it may or may not benefit the client to use the product we sell, the main ethical issue is whether we are unfairly using the power of the therapeutic relationship. Is the client really free to say "No"? Or would she want to make a purchase to please us?

Also, selling anything to a client other than the professional services we have contracted for creates a dual relationship and dual relationships are problematic. (See Chapter Nine on Dual Relationships.) Suppose the client has an allergic reaction to the algae the practitioner sold her or just didn't obtain as much benefit from taking it as she had hoped? It could damage their working relationship.

Many of the practitioners interviewed for this book expressed alarm at the growing number of multilevel marketing ventures with which manual therapists are involved. They question whether the practice, perhaps unwittingly, takes advantage of clients' positive transference and general good will toward their practitioners. They express concern that the main focus is on the well-being of the practitioner's finances and not the well-being of the therapeutic relationship. If clients are interested in a particular product, then we can refer them to someone else. In this situation there is no harm, as long as we don't benefit financially from the referral or talk clients into trying the product.

Is it ever ethical to sell a product to a client? If the clients' needs are put first and it's a service to them, it may be a clean exchange. For example, a chiropractor colleague has orthopedic pillows on hand that he sells, at cost, to his clients who need them. He sells them as a convenience to his clients, rather than for his own benefit. Also, he doesn't try to influence them to buy pillows.

Refusing to Work with a Client or Stopping Work with a Client: The Ethical Standard

We have a right to refuse to work with a prospective client or to refuse to continue working with a client if we think that a professional environment cannot be maintained. If something the client is doing is disrespectful, or if there is some reason we cannot form a positive alliance, we should not work with that client.

Refusing to Work with a Client or Stopping Work with a Client: Judgment Calls

> Your regular client arrives, having spent the afternoon doing yard work, and is uncharacteristically dirty and sweaty.

> You have worked with a couple on outcall basis several times. While you are alone with the husband, he makes suggestive remarks.

> You weigh 100 pounds. Your prospective client weighs twice that and asks for deep work.

There are many reasons we may choose not to work with a client. Some massage therapy clinics post a sign and/or have clients read a statement which says they can refuse to work with someone or terminate work because of the client's poor hygiene or because of inappropriate sexual behavior or comments. There are other reasons a client may not be appropriate for our work or may be beyond our abilities—they may be mentally ill or they may have physical conditions that are contraindicated by the kind of work we do.

We don't need to take on clients with physical or emotional problems that overwhelm us. We may want to limit the number of clients with special difficulties whom we see. We may want to limit the clients who take extra energy in terms of phone calls and consultations outside the session, for whatever reason. Some psychotherapists, for instance, don't treat more than one suicidal patient at a time. Massage therapists may want to limit the number of clients with whom they have difficulty working—for instance, very large or very densely muscled clients or clients who are in acute and distressing pain. We need to know what the limits of our skill and our physical abilities are; it's unethical to knowingly take on a client we cannot serve well.

In the first situation above, I would guess that most practitioners wouldn't mind working with an occasionally grimy client—such as the one who came in from yard work. Those who do mind need to make their policies clear up front to avoid the embarrassment of turning away a client.

In the case of the husband who made inappropriate remarks, if someone has made offensive or degrading remarks, we shouldn't work with him. (It's different when a regular client makes a sexually-oriented joke that is clearly not meant to be disrespectful, and we aren't offended.) The husband could be given a warning that we won't continue working with him unless he stops being suggestive. If he continues, it would be best to refuse to work with him, even though we might lose the wife's business too. (The question of what, if anything, to tell the wife will be discussed under Confidentiality below.)

We also don't need to take on clients who tax our physical capacities. We can be straightforward about our reasons: "I can't do justice to someone your size. May I give you the names of some practitioners who would be more appropriate?"

Sometimes we may want to decline to work with a difficult client because we ourselves are in an unstable time. A bodyworker reports:

> During a time while I was under personal stress, a man with whom I was casually acquainted wanted to begin working with me. He was suffering from an undiagnosed, mysterious illness that was causing alarming symptoms of weakness and debilitation. I could tell that he would need extra reassurance and support during this frightening time. Because of my own stress level, I referred him to a colleague who was in better shape at the time.

When we decline to work with someone, for whatever reasons, we want to do it without judgment and without room for argument. A good statement is, "I'm just not comfortable working with you." We can put the responsibility on ourselves.

Confidentiality: The Ethical Standard

Anything that a client says or does, any information we have about a client cannot be revealed unless disclosure is required by law or court order or is absolutely necessary for the protection of the public. Instances when we can legally breach confidentiality include situations in which there is: a threat to self or others, suspicion of child abuse or a medical emergency.*

Confidentiality: Judgment Calls

In the earlier situation of the husband who was sexually inappropriate, what do you say to his wife if you decide not to work with him? She is your client also, and you've been scheduling their appointments back to back at their home.

It's a good idea to make sure that new clients know we are bound by confidentiality: it may be a concern, and they may not be aware of our standards of practice. This is especially true if we know the client in another context, if we know someone that the client knows or if the client is a well-known person in our community. It can also help deflect any problems that arise. For example, in the above situation, the standards of confidentiality dictate that we can't tell the wife why we have stopped seeing her husband. We cannot even imply or suggest. We have to say, "I know that this is your husband, but I can't ethically talk about another client." If we've told her about our standards at the outset, it makes reinforcing the policy easier.

If we have clients who know each other, we cannot talk about one to the other. If our client Susan knows that her friend Tom

---

*Federal confidentiality law—part two, CFR, #42

is a new client, she may fish for information. "Boy, Tom's really tight, isn't he?" or "I hope he's dealing with his problems at work." If we respond to such comments with any information about Tom, we not only violate his confidentiality, we damage our relationship with Susan. If we talk about Tom to her, what prevents us from talking to Tom or others about *her*?

What about revealing that someone is a client? Psychotherapists cannot do that, according to their standards. Although it's not been clear that this is a rule for manual therapists, it's a very good idea and can be a part of maintaining confidentiality. There is no legitimate need to tell a third party that someone is a client and doing so risks offending the client.

Quite often, if a client has referred a friend who then becomes our client, we thank the referrer, thereby letting him know that his friend is now a client. While that's a common practice and seems harmless and also good business manners to express gratitude, we might want to re-think it. Doesn't it violate that friend's privacy? Or a client says, "I told Joe about you. Did he ever call?" We want to thank the client for making the referral, but we don't have to reveal whether Joe ever called or not. Just because the client made a referral, Joe's interactions with us don't become his business. We can say, "I understand why you want to know, but I don't want to reveal what may be private for someone else." Or we can ask, when we first talk with a prospective client, if he's okay with our thanking his friend for the referral.

What do we do when we have to leave a message for a client at home or at the office? We can't identify ourselves as "his massage therapist" or "her polarity therapist" unless we have the client's permission. It's safest to ask, during the first session,

"How would you like me to identify myself if I need to leave you a message?"

Sometimes it's tempting to name-drop when a person who is well-known or famous is or has been a client. There are no exceptions to confidentiality. Famous people appreciate their privacy and have a right to it. Name-dropping is rarely impressive and only reveals us as practitioners who don't safeguard clients' privacy.

Respecting confidentiality also means that treatment rooms should be sound-proofed so that people walking by the door can't overhear the talk during a session. Likewise, we need to keep our client records or insurance papers out of sight, including signed checks from the day's clients. A colleague expressed distress over seeing another practitioner's client records lying about in a waiting room, accessible to anyone. Receptionists also need to understand that clients' names and their reasons for coming are confidential.

Amrita Daigle, Trager Approach instructor, has noted that it can be difficult to maintain confidentiality unless we have a legitimate outlet for the feelings that build up in us during the work week. We need a way to deal with the emotional stories that people tell us and the stresses we face. Daigle suggests that we find a healthy outlet for our feelings, such as drawing, dancing or meditating and use it regularly. Supervisors are also excellent and appropriate outlets. (We should let new clients know that we sometimes discuss our work with a supervisor who is also bound by confidentiality and get their permission to do so.) Getting ongoing bodywork also helps with emotional overload.

Other Ethical Standards and Implementation

Some ethics guidelines are fairly straightforward: we just need help with implementing them.

False Claims: The Ethical Standard

Making false claims or inflated promises is unethical. It's unethical to obtain clients by persuasion or influence, or to use comments that contain untrue statements. It is unethical to create inflated or unjustified expectations of favorable results.

False Claims: Implementation

In describing our work to a prospective client, we need to be honest about its limits and also any possible negative side effects. We can never guarantee a result. We can speak of the benefits that we know to be true. For instance, we can say (assuming that it's true to the best of our knowledge) that "many people" feel less tension, fewer aches and pains or whatever. We can state that "many people" have experienced alleviation of general symptoms. We need to be careful about subtly or blatantly leading the client to expect specific cures or fixes. Promising to fix a specific problem is dangerous. The causes of physical problems are complex and the outcome of our treatments can't be predicted. A colleague says:

> Anytime I've done an oversell about the benefits of my method of bodywork, it comes back to haunt me. My reasons are usually well-intentioned. Sometimes, I'm tempted to do a "hard sell" because I really like a prospective client and *want* to be able to help him. I believe strongly in my work and sometimes that makes me promise too much. I think it always

backfires on me. That client is always the one who doesn't get any relief from the treatment.

Scope of Practice: The Ethical Standard

The dangers of exceeding our scope of practice have been discussed in Chapter Two. It's unethical to represent ourselves as having training or expertise that we do not have, such as suggesting that we are skilled in handling serious medical conditions.

We have an obligation to refer clients to appropriately trained professionals and, with the client's permission, to consult with the other professionals who are treating our client. Some practitioners take this a step further and refuse to see a seriously ill client unless the client gives permission to consult with their primary practitioner.

Scope of Practice: Implementation

Practitioners who exceed the scope of their practice were a cause of concern for many of the people I interviewed. Some people claim to work with emotional and psychological issues who have had no training or supervision. One weekend workshop (or even a few) doesn't make an expert in physical manipulations—cranial work, visceral manipulation or whatever else that's popular. It's unethical to advertise ourselves, on our business cards or verbally, as proficient in a method for which we have only a superficial knowledge or training.

If a method is relatively well-known, such as Rolfing, there are always untrained people eager to jump on the bandwagon:

> Presenting a Rolfing lecture and demonstration to a group of massage therapists, I was taken aback when one therapist raised her hand

and said, "When *I* rolf people, they always throw up." This woman had never received a single session from a Certified Rolfer, much less attended a legitimate training, and had only the most superficial idea of what the work was, erroneously thinking that any deep manipulation is Rolfing. She also didn't know that it is illegal to claim to be "Rolfing" without the proper credentials (as it is for all trademarked and servicemarked methods).

We need to respect the time and training it takes to become a manual therapist of a certain school, a psychologist, cranial osteopath, medical doctor, chiropractor or whatever. And at the same time, we need to respect the value of our own skills. Dianne Polseno, ethics columnist for the *Massage Therapy Journal*, says of massage therapy and bodywork, "We are better at what we do than any other health care professional. Other professionals say 'Tell us what your hands feel.' That's the gift we bring—what we feel under our hands."

We are unique as health care professionals in the amount of time we spend with our clients and the level of attention and care we give them. There is plenty of healing in simply being with people in a conscious, attentive way—listening to them, listening to their bodies. If we appreciate the strength and value of our own work, we won't feel the need to pad our resumes.

When we don't have the expertise—the psychological or medical training to help a client—we are obligated to refer them to an appropriate practitioner, or at least let them know that another kind of practitioner might be of more benefit.

Informed Consent: The Ethical Standard

We need to have clients' informed consent for (1) the basic treatment or kind of manual therapy that we offer, (2) any work that is near clients' genitals or anus or a woman's breasts, (3) any work that is near an area that we know to be sensitive or triggering for a particular client and (4) any work that is different from the work we've contracted to do.

This means that clients know both the possible benefits and the possible side effects of our work. For instance, they may need to be told that when the body is healing naturally, sometimes clients feel worse before they feel better. Clients also need to know the reasons for a specific treatment or why we need to work in a sensitive area.

Informed Consent: Implementation

Some practitioners obtain written consent from new clients before they begin work. They use a form that explains what the general benefits of the work are and also assures the client that there are no guarantees, that no medical treatment or diagnosis is involved, etc. Having a client sign such a form is excellent protection for the practitioner also. Although it may not hold up in court as a legal document, it can be a deterrent to lawsuits.

In an intake interview, clients should also be told, either in writing or verbally, about any contraindications. As we are working, we need to explain and get agreement for any work that is potentially threatening, such as work near the genitals. If we decide to use a different method with the client, other than what has been agreed upon, we need to explain that method and get the client's consent.

A key to the idea of consent is that, because of transference, clients are not as free to say "no" as they would ordinarily be. This is true especially if they are already on the table and could be in an altered state. We need to be clear with clients that they can ask us to stop or refuse a treatment at any time.

Disrespect of Other Professionals: The Ethical Standard
It's unethical to imply that our skill level or our method of manual therapy is superior to either another practitioner's or another kind of work.

Disrespect of Other Professionals: Implementation
When we malign another practitioner, it makes us look insecure in our client's eyes. If we make critical remarks about the practitioner the client is seeing or has seen, it can sound as if we're being critical of the client's judgment. We want to avoid careless talk, gossip, personal remarks, or assessments about the competence of another practitioner. We all have ex-clients who think we're skilled and compassionate and those who do not. We want to take care with another practitioner's reputation.

The same goes for maligning other kinds of manual therapies or alternative health practices or being disrespectful of the medical profession. It just makes us look small and can offend clients loyal to that kind of treatment.

Staying Out of Trouble:
The Therapeutic Relationship
Ethics is about relationships. That means we can follow all the laws and still get into trouble. Most ethics complaints and lawsuits have little to do with the practitioner's incompetence or departure from strict adherence to ethical guidelines, and a good deal to do with the relationship between the client and the practitioner.

A study published in a medical journal showed that doctors were more likely to be sued if their patients felt they were rushing visits, not answering questions or being rude in some other way. A comparison between doctors who had often been sued and those who had not showed no difference in the competence level of the two groups as perceived by their colleagues. However, the ones who had never been sued were more likely to be seen by their patients as concerned, accessible and willing to communicate.

The administrator for a bodywork association who fields complaints against its members reinforces the need to be accessible and willing to communicate. She says that quite often bodyworkers will stonewall a complaining client and that they could avoid having a complaint lodged against them if they would simply answer the client's phone calls and allow grievances to be aired. Unless clients are abusive or harassing, the best thing we can do, even if we feel we committed no error, is allow them to speak their minds and let them know that we regret their dissatisfaction.

Clients have to be upset or angry in order to file a complaint. Assuming that the practitioner practices in a normally ethical way, clients' anger may come from feeling that the practitioner has been indifferent to their feelings and/or emotionally abandoned them in some way. Or the practitioner may have been lacking in compassion or failed to show interest in or listen to them.

The fact that ethics is grounded in the therapeutic relationship is all the more reason not to work with those about whom we have predominantly negative feelings. And it's all the more reason to have regular supervision to help smooth out relationships with our clients.

Bending Boundaries

The "therapeutic relationship" is defined by framework and boundaries. What seems like a small exception in our framework can be a warning sign that we're headed down a dangerous path by leaving the boundaries of the therapeutic relationship. We need to give careful thought to any changes that we make—coming in earlier or later than usual, charging less than we ordinarily do, giving a client a gift, working in some way that we don't usually. The phrase, "I don't usually do this, but..." should set off alarms in our heads.

Wanting to bend our boundaries or change our regular framework for a client is a red flag. We don't want to be influenced by a client or by our (not necessarily romantic) feelings about a client to depart from our usual professional stance. Once we step outside the boundaries of the therapeutic relationship, we invite trouble.

> A male practitioner was touched by the story of a new female client working her way through school who said she didn't have the financial resources to pay his usual fee. She was also engaging and attractive, and although he wasn't sexually attracted to her, he found her appealing. He agreed to see her at a discount. He also sometimes changed his schedule to suit her class schedule.
>
> As the months went by, there were signs that she had more money available than she had

indicated—she would talk of taking vacations to the beach or buying a new television. He finally confronted her with this and asked her to pay the regular fee. She said she was insulted and didn't come back to him as a client. Later, he found out that she had developed a crush on him and, perhaps feeling rejected by him, was telling people in the community that he had made sexual advances toward her.

Some practitioners will make exceptions for long-term clients that they have come to trust—letting them defer payment, for example. Making an exception for someone who has been a conscientious client for several years isn't generally the same problem as making an exception for a new client.

Beware "The Rescue"

Making special exceptions for a client is often motivated by a wish to "rescue" the client in a way that's not healthy. What makes a rescue unhealthy is the underlying idea—if there is no real basis for the idea—that the client can't be held to the usual demands and restrictions we place on other clients. An unhealthy rescue would involve, for instance, giving a financial discount to an able-bodied person who is free to seek gainful employment. On the other hand, a healthy rescue might be giving a discount to a student, an elderly person on a fixed income or a person with a serious illness. (Such discounts still have to be monitored. See Chapter Eight on money issues.)

Here are signs of an unhealthy rescue:

- Feeling a little (or a good deal) manipulated. We may be responding to a "guilt trip."

- Feeling trapped into working with this person on his/her terms.
- Feeling that we are the only person who can work with this person.
- Wanting to be seen as nice.
- Being afraid (sometimes without realizing it) of the client's anger if he doesn't get his way.

Unhealthy rescues involve putting a client in a special category; they involve thinking that the client is too inadequate, too busy, too precious, etc. to be held within the usual boundaries. They are based on a subtle kind of disrespect for the client ("They just can't handle it.") and will always backfire.

In the above story about the male practitioner and the student, because the client was a student, the practitioner did have some basis for giving her a discount. However, there's also the possibility that he was motivated by wanting to please a charming young woman and have her see him as a hero or "good guy." His judgment may have been clouded.

We invite problems when we are involved in an unhealthy rescue. Clients don't feel thoroughly safe in an environment where they don't know what the boundaries are; they then can lose respect for us as professionals and can attack our professional status.

Also, when a new client wants many exceptions made for him, we want to be careful with that client. Assuming that we run our practices in ethical ways, if someone is going to sue us, it will likely be someone who is mentally disturbed. Often, emotionally ill or confused people balk at our regular framework and will ask for exceptions from the start. Giving in to them in the beginning, even in small ways, can snowball into major problems.

When There Are No Warning Signs: The Need for Documentation and Professional Association

I've heard of instances of practitioners being sued or complained against where there were no significant warning signs.* What saved them in court was that they had carefully documented the client's presenting problems and course of treatment. We need to keep careful notes, especially when we feel unease about a client, when we work with medical issues and when we work with clients with abuse issues. The importance of documentation cannot be stressed enough.

The other factor that was helpful to these practitioners was their belonging to a recognized and respected professional group. The client's attorneys will want to make a manual therapy practitioner look sinister, dishonest or fly-by-night. Belonging to a respected national group will enhance the practitioner's image. In addition, professional associations will often provide witnesses to back up the legitimacy of our methods.

The Right Thing

What's right may vary depending on the client and the situation. How strictly do we interpret the guideline, for instance, that it's not ethical to benefit personally from a client? No one is going to haul us into court if we have cleverly placed our dying ficus plant in the middle of the room, hoping our next client, a regular of many years and owner of a plant shop, will notice it and give us good advice. If the plant shop owner was

---

*Individual circumstances of ethics complaints will vary. Practitioners who have been officially complained against or threatened with a lawsuit should consult an attorney and also work closely with the ethics boards of their organizations.

a new client and we met him at the door with a barrage of questions about our ailing flora, again, we probably wouldn't be sued, but we might lose him as a client or at least, make him uneasy.

The main consideration when making ethics decisions is whether an action will harm the client and/or the therapeutic relationship. As the manual therapies become increasingly popular, we will have increased opportunities to use our new power and strength in ways that take advantage of clients or in ways that benefit them.

Sexual Issues: Protecting Our Clients

Chapter Six

Our work can be a sacred calling. Some practitioners see massage therapy, bodywork and movement education as ways to heal the soul and enliven the spirit. Many are led to this work for high-minded reasons. Ah, but then there's the messiness of dealing with the flesh.

Sometimes clients are sexually attracted to their practitioners, sometimes practitioners are sexually attracted to their clients. (Probably no more than, say, the average hardware store clerk, but still, it happens.) Crushes flourish, and confusion abounds. Many massage therapists are still contending with a portion of the public that thinks "massage" means prostitution.

The honest pleasure of sensuality is part of the profession, which means that the dark possibilities of seduction and exploitation are lurking in the background. Sexuality is a basic and potentially overwhelming element of our work—how do we deal with it?

Can We Talk?

To begin with, we need to start talking honestly with each other. Sexual issues are the most emotionally charged and least talked about issues in the manual therapies. And because there's not enough dialogue, we don't learn from one another's experiences.

True, we do talk about blatant and obvious problems—clients who think we're prostitutes or practitioners who habitually become sexually involved with clients. These are important issues to discuss, but there is a wider range, a gray area that needs exploring also.

When I started researching this book, I was surprised at how complex and painful the stories were from both clients and practitioners. I heard stories of well-meaning and presumably well-trained practitioners who had stumbled into tangled, destructive situations that might have been avoided had they known the warning signs and responded to them.

- A client thinks that a woman practitioner who is working close to her genitals is sexually violating her.
- A bodyworker becomes sexually involved with a client and only later sees how damaging the relationship was to the client.
- A massage therapist ends sessions by kissing female clients on the forehead, not realizing how this seemingly small gesture can be invasive and even traumatizing.

The emotions about these stories run deep for both client and practitioner. Even if falsely accused of violating a client, a practitioner's distress is long-lasting. And the effect on the client when sexual boundaries are crossed, whether intentional or not, is particularly damaging because of the power difference between client and practitioner.

The Generic Erection

When I was trained as a massage therapist in the late '70s, there was little mention of sexual issues as they relate to clients.

I remember one useful bit of insight, offered by my Swedish massage teacher: "When a man gets an erection, it may just be like a dog wagging his tail."

She was saying that an erection can be nothing more than an automatic physical response to intimate touch and that the client did not necessarily feel interest or disrespect toward the massage therapist. She also added, "If it makes you uncomfortable, don't try to pretend it doesn't. Have him turn over on his stomach."

Those are interesting pieces of advice. But considering the sensuality that often accompanies bodywork, the intimacy of it and the general confusion about sexual boundaries in this culture, it wasn't nearly enough. These days there's more awareness and discussion in schools about handling sexual feelings, both those of the practitioner and those of the client, but probably still not enough.

Perhaps in an attempt to overcome the image that some people have of "massage" as a euphemism for prostitution, many massage schools initially seemed to move to an opposing stance, all but ignoring the sexual components of our work. Also, many manual therapy schools seemed to copy the traditional medical model of education, which downplays all aspects of the relationship between client and practitioner, including sexuality.

For whatever reason, in spite of the fact that we work in an intimate situation that involves putting our hands on people wearing little or no clothing, manual therapy practitioners have often acted as if all sexuality stays politely parked outside the door.

Boundary Confusion

It's testimony to the good intentions and good sense of most practitioners that there don't seem to be more instances of sexual misconduct. (Rumors of alleged sexual misconduct travel quickly, yet rarely have I heard such stories about other practitioners.) But we sometimes forget how suggestive and confusing the situation can be. Not only are we touching people who are naked or close to it, but our work invites them to enter an altered state that leaves them open and vulnerable to us and also to the memories buried in their tissue.

Many people have been sexually abused as children—the client may have been abused and the practitioner may have been abused. Therefore, either one or both can come into the session with a distorted sense of appropriate sexual boundaries.

Clients who have been sexually abused can be hyper-alert to signs of danger or seduction and therefore more likely to misread a careless word or gesture. At the same time, they can be blind to a truly dangerous situation when a therapist is being inappropriate. Practitioners who have a history of childhood sexual abuse can make the same mistakes: they can assume that a client has sexual intentions when he does not; they can fail to respond adequately when a client actually *is* being offensive. Practitioners who have been sexually abused may also be unable to see their own seductiveness or inappropriateness with a client. Boundary violations may unconsciously feel comfortable and familiar to them.

Even without a history of sexual abuse, sex can be a highly charged emotional issue. Unless we have worked with our own issues both in therapy and in supervision, we probably have blind spots about them. For clients, the potential for them to mistrust us or misread our intentions is increased by the fact that we have credentials that are often unfamiliar to the public and that some of us work out of our homes, in what is actually a converted bedroom.

In order for our clients to feel safe, we need to define the situation as professional by providing clear boundaries and a stable framework. We are touching people, often with a tenderness and gentle attentiveness similar to a lover's. Like lovers, sometimes we blend with clients, so that it's hard to tell where one person stops and the other starts; there is a sense of merging. When the professional boundaries are clear, it can be wonderfully healing for the client. When they aren't, it can be harmful or even disastrous.

There are lessons to learn from the stories about sexual boundary confusion that I heard from other practitioners. One is that such incidences are much more common than we think. Confusion is bred in silence—if we can begin to talk more frankly, we will learn from one another rather than each of us learning alone through painful experience.

Another lesson from these stories is that when practitioners have unwittingly crossed a sexual boundary or have been perceived as crossing one, they have often ignored warning signs and disregarded red flags along the way. The next section gives some guidelines that may help us recognize those signs.

This chapter isn't intended as a comprehensive guide to the subject of sexual issues or working with sexually abused clients. There are books written for manual therapists on these subjects and specific trainings offered. Refer to Related Readings for books.

We will always have clients who have been sexually abused. Even if these clients are not consciously working with abuse issues, it's a good idea for us to be educated about the subject. However, any practitioner working with a client actively dealing with sexual abuse issues needs to have outside supervision from a knowledgeable professional. Such clients should be referred to psychotherapists if they're not already in treatment.

Silence Isn't Agreement

Sometimes practitioners unconsciously stumble across sexual boundaries—flirting with a client, not realizing that even hugging a client can be violating or being attracted to a client. It's confusing territory that most of us need help navigating.

Clients usually won't tell us directly when we make them uncomfortable. This is especially true when their discomfort is around a sexual issue.

> A successful businesswoman receiving a massage in a spa thought that the practitioner was working too close to her genitals. She didn't think the massage therapist, an older Asian woman, was making sexual advances, but she was still uncomfortable. In the business world, this woman had a diplomatic but straightforward style of dealing with people and expressed her feelings easily. In the role of client, she said nothing. But she never went back to that therapist.

Even if the client is an acquaintance or colleague, even if the person is usually assertive in the outside world, once in the role of client, she or he can have a hard time saying, "no."

A client's silence doesn't always mean agreement. We all act differently when we're naked, or partially so, with "an expert" looming over us. We usually do not feel the freedom to defend or assert ourselves in the ways we would in a social encounter.

It helps clients voice their feelings if we demonstrate in many ways our interest in hearing how they feel and what they have to say. Bill Scholl, a Trager instructor, makes sure he asks clients to let him know if anything makes them uncomfortable. He does this even if he has worked with them many times before. We never know what someone is bringing into a session. We need to let clients know that they can always ask us to stop what we're doing, even if they do not have a "rational" reason and even if they feel they're being rude by doing so.

Quicksand and Minefields

Any practitioner, male or female, gay or straight, can be accused of sexually violating a client. Seductive or careless practitioners are not the only ones accused. Even good-hearted, conscientious practitioners can have clients misread their intentions.

Any client can misinterpret the intentions of any practitioner. Heterosexual women practitioners can be accused by heterosexual women clients, for instance. Sexual abuse and violation issues are about power and they cross all lines of gender and sexual orientation. The body holds the unconscious and the unconscious is often primitive and irrational. That's why we have to provide clear boundaries when we do this work.

A heterosexual female practitioner was working around a female client's sacrum and was suddenly accused by the client of violating her anally. The practitioner was horrified and immediately removed her hands from the client. She worked the rest of the session to calm the client's concerns, but the client never seemed to regain trust in her and stopped coming for sessions.

In retrospect, the practitioner realized she might have avoided the misunderstanding if she'd taken more care. She was doing deep emotionally-oriented work, and she knew this client was fragile and confused about boundaries. She most likely could have avoided the misunderstanding if the client had not been naked—if she had asked her client to leave on her underwear or had worked on top of the draping.

She also should have gotten the informed consent of the client: during the session, she could have explained where she wanted to work and the purpose of working in that area and then asked the client's permission.

No one is immune to being misunderstood by a client. However, if we consistently attend to framework and boundaries, we'll be more likely to head off trouble from the start. I've heard many stories, some about false accusations, some about true abuse—either way, practitioners usually made subtle boundary mistakes long before they ever got into deeper trouble. Three conditions in which boundary mistakes thrive are specialness, secrets and dual relationships.

Specialness

"Specialness," even when the emotions seem positive, is always a red flag. Being overwhelmed with attraction to a client or intensely identifying with a client is different from having compassion for or even loving our clients. In the therapeutic relationship, this can be traumatizing:

> A woman related that during the course of seeing a female bodyworker for many months, she developed an intense transference—she was deeply infatuated with her practitioner. She also felt that the practitioner was very drawn to her and that the practitioner had lost her objectivity. The relationship developed into an inappropriate situation where, under the guise of therapy, the therapist had touched the client's breasts and genitals during several sessions. The client ended up feeling emotionally and physically seduced and damaged. Her confused feelings of shame and guilt were so powerful that she had never before discussed this relationship with anyone. She was only able to discuss it with me in response to an online questionnaire, where she could remain totally anonymous.

Although we don't know what the internal dynamics were for this practitioner, what happened to make her use such poor judgment, it's obvious that the client became very special to her in a way that wasn't professional or healthy. The client said that both she and the bodyworker were dealing with issues related to their childhood sexual abuse. (And this indicates a boundary was crossed early on when the practitioner shared her personal story.) Perhaps the therapist began to identify so strongly with this particular client that she lost her sense of boundaries and appropriateness. She may have been duplicating her own childhood abuse with this client—exploiting a vulnerable person just as she had been exploited as a child.

Specialness is also a red flag when we feel "special" as a practitioner. Thinking we are the only ones who can work with a particular client or save her or fully bring out her potential are warning signals that our judgment is off.

When we start having such inappropriate and strong feelings about clients, we need to get outside help. When we start wanting to bend boundaries with a client—for instance, to share personal information more than we normally would—we need to discuss our feelings with a supervisor or counselor. There is nothing wrong with having such feelings and it could be that our impulses are just fine, but we need to know how to keep the relationship focused on what is best for the client. We should talk it over with an objective and trusted professional with training in human dynamics. If the decision is to refer the client to another professional, that should be done carefully so that it's not injurious to the client.

No matter how seductive the client or how equal we feel the relationship is, the practitioner is responsible for keeping good boundaries. Our relationships with clients are never equal and we can damage our clients if we act on inappropriate feelings. When clients are "in love with" us or have crushes on us, those feelings can be part of a positive therapeutic experience, if boundaries are kept.

We need to know enough about ourselves to stay objective and neither step on clients' feelings nor exploit their vulnerability. Supervision can help us understand the dynamics. Seductive clients, for instance, are not asking for us to be their lovers; they're telling us how they habitually deal with power in relationships. They're telling us how they usually get into trouble in their lives or how they get attention. Supervision can help us turn the experience into a healthy, learning one for both us and our clients.

Secrets

In the online story involving the two women, there was probably another red flag—secrecy. I doubt that this bodyworker shared with other bodyworkers the details of her work with the client. We're headed for trouble anytime we are doing something with a client, or even having a feeling about a client, that we want to keep secret or that we would not share with our colleagues.

When we feel that desire for secrecy, we need to share our situation with a supervisor or teacher, as hard as it may be to do. It could be that there's no reason for us to feel uncomfortable. Or it could be that we need help with the client before it turns into an even more difficult problem.

Too Many Hats

Another way we can get into a troubled relationship with clients is by having dual relationships. In a dual relationship, the boundaries are already blurred. Working with people who we know in some other way, doing trades or working with people who share a community with us, can often lead to confusion about sexual boundaries. We would think that the more someone knows us, the less chance that they would misread our intentions. However, the opposite is often true. Here's how the dynamic of transference affected a trade between two colleagues:

> Sally, a massage therapist who was sexually abused by her father, agreed to do a trade with Jim for sessions in his form of emotionally-oriented bodywork. As the trade went on, the work she was getting from Jim brought up her feelings about the abuse. As the client, she began to look on Jim as a father figure.
>
> To fulfill her side of the trade, she gave Jim a massage every other week. He was naked, she was touching him. There were just too many boundaries crossed. As Jim worked near her breasts in one session, she confused an incest memory with the present reality and decided that Jim was trying to seduce her. They talked it out, but the trust was never the same and the trade was terminated.

Trades make it difficult to maintain clear and clean boundaries. Practitioners doing emotionally-oriented work or deep transformational work should never do trades. The confusion of dual relationships makes trades potentially harmful.

The same confusion can occur if we are working with someone who is part of a "family" group that we're in—we are both serious students of the same yoga teacher, we're in the same Buddhist sangha or are members of the same church. When we're working with such a person, we need to be alert to the negative transference about "family" that can get projected onto us because of our association with that group: not everyone has good memories of family. Even though the Buddhist (or whatever kind of) group that we belong to may be spiritual and well-intentioned, our client may have buried in his unconscious the idea that "family" means abuse, and we may get the brunt of that.

Dual relationships are discussed further in Chapter Nine.

Crushes

It's normal for clients to develop crushes on their practitioners. People bring all kinds of tender longings, old hurts and broken hearts to their sessions. And there we are—the picture of kindliness, warmth and selfless giving. We seem to be the perfect parent/friend/confidante they have always wanted.

When these feelings are aroused in clients, there's usually a sexual component to them, as well. The mistake is for us to think those feelings are about us, or that they are the same as grown-up feelings of wanting a sexual relationship. They are not. If we understand where crushes come from, we can understand how damaging it would be to try to initiate a sexual relationship with the client.

Crushes can come from a very young stage in the client's emotional development. They may be feelings that were unresolved at an early age—wanting to be loved unconditionally, wanting to be just like Dad or Mom, wanting a parent's approval.

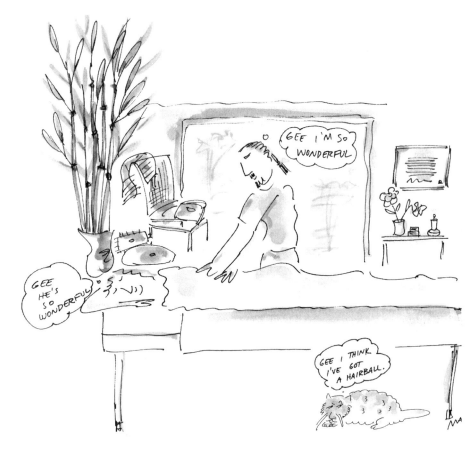

Our clients allow those longings to come up because they think they're safe, and that we won't exploit them.

Crushes need to be treated as a sign of the client's trust. We can't let them go to our heads. It's very flattering to have someone wide-eyed over us, hanging on our every word and laughing at all our jokes. We have to remember that it's a projection of a deep longing, and that it says more about the client than it does about us. Gentle care should be taken with the vulnerability of a client with a crush.

Dating An Ex-Client

Surely we all know not to have sex with a client or to date someone who is our client. But can we date an ex-client? The answer is that it depends. It depends on the professional relationship, the intensity of the transference, how emotionally stable the client is, how emotionally stable the practitioner is and how much time has lapsed since the therapeutic work. The most important element is whether the transference and countertransference issues are resolved, and that's a complex question.

The point for practitioners is not to take advantage of the power given us by our role. With some clients, we could never have a social, and therefore certainly not a sexual, relationship. For others, it might work. If the situation is that of a bodyworker in a health spa who saw a client once for an athletic massage, it's more likely that a strong transference didn't develop. On the other hand, practitioners of emotionally-oriented work that evokes deep transference should give serious consideration before beginning to date an ex-client. The possibility of their taking advantage of a client's transference is strong. Also, by doing so, a practitioner who dates an ex-client opens himself up to scrutiny by his colleagues and professional associations.

A client who comes to a practitioner in crisis or terrible pain may perceive that practitioner as the hero on the white horse. A practitioner who is able to provide relief from pain when all other methods have failed will always seem larger than life to that client. If there are any elements that enhance the practitioner's stature in the eyes of the client, the relationship will have trouble achieving equal footing; there is likely a strong transference, which makes a social relationship difficult.

Many manual therapy associations say that dating a client may be OK if you wait several months after ending the professional relationship. Others never allow it. Practitioners need to check with the licensing laws in their states and the ethical guidelines of the professional organizations to which they belong.

The reason for delaying social interaction after concluding the therapeutic relationship is to make sure that neither the client nor the practitioner is still caught up in the rosy glow of transference/countertransference. There needs to be time for reality to have set in. Whether to date an ex-client isn't a decision to make lightly. It can damage a practitioner's reputation, and if other clients know about the relationship, it can interfere with their work. The safest solution is never to date ex-clients.

> A client with a crush on his bodyworker asked her for a date. Because she was able to honestly say that she never dates ex-clients, he was able to save face and continue his professional relationship with her. Suppose she had refused him and he knew of other ex-clients she had dated? Suppose she had accepted, had developed a relationship with him and it had ended in quarrels?

> In another situation, a male practitioner turned down a client's invitation for a date. The client knew that wasn't always his policy, that he had dated other clients, and she ended up feeling so hurt that she stopped going to him professionally.

"Special" feelings, intense feelings about clients are indications of countertransference. Feeling that a client is different from the others, wanting to rush into dating him, thinking that others wouldn't understand the "special" feelings the two of you have are all warning signs. When there is that adolescent sense that the intensity of the attraction justifies breaking the rules, it's a red flag. It's best to talk it out with a colleague, mentor, and/or supervisor who is nonjudgmental. (All professionals are vulnerable to attractions to clients. A supervisor or mentor should know that by talking about, rather than acting on the attraction, the practitioner is being professional and appropriate.)

The Error of Sexualizing Our Work

The more we can keep clear boundaries between our social lives and our work lives in place, the happier we will be. Also, we will be avoiding danger zones and protecting our reputations. Working with people to whom we're attracted can blur the edges of what we're doing. We're sexualizing our work if we're trying to get to know someone as both a new client and as a dating prospect. Our work needs to be about the client and not about our social needs. We can't have it both ways. (This question was discussed in depth in Chapter Five on ethical issues.)

Another red flag that we're sexualizing our work is wearing seductive clothes all the time or for one particular client. Short shorts, tank tops and cleavage are for the beach. When our work life begins to look like our dating life, it's time to get supervision and/or therapy. We're only human and we can't always sort these issues out on our own.

Other Cautions

There are a number of other areas where it makes sense to be cautious, to think of the potential for misinterpretation by a vulnerable client.

Comments about the client's body: We need to choose our words carefully even when saying positive things about a client's body. Even "Why do you criticize your body? You look great!" can sound personal or suggestive. Sometimes we want to compliment a client because we see that he or she has a negative body image and we want to help. However, we're probably better off avoiding all comments about how we think the client's body looks aesthetically. It could be heard as a sexual comment and making such a remark also assumes that we're experts in evaluating how bodies should look—which we are not. It's just one more way that we can keep ourselves humble by not pretending to know more than the client.

Draping: I can't think of any instance where draping would be a bad idea. In most massage licensing, it's the law. For deep work or emotional work, having a client wear underwear is a must, in addition to draping. When in doubt, go for more cover, rather than less. It's respectful to the client's privacy and a way to protect ourselves from misunderstandings.

Undressing: Clients need to dress and undress in private and they also need to know that they do not have to undress at all if it makes them uncomfortable. Let them know that they can wear a bathing suit or whatever else is suitable—for instance, athletic shorts, and a comfortable bra or tank top. Be sure that clients really understand that it's fine for them to wear as much clothing as they need to feel comfortable.

Locked doors: The question of whether or not the door was locked has been a crucial point in some court cases in which a practitioner was sued for sexual harassment. Even if the client isn't locked in and could unlock the door himself, the point is whether the client could quickly and easily leave the room. In many situations, a practitioner may want to lock the door to protect the client from unwanted intrusion—a stranger wandering into an office by mistake. A cautious way to handle that would be to explain our reasons for wanting to lock the door and give clients the option of locked or unlocked.

Intrusive work: Some manual therapies can involve intrusive work. If we have good reason to work in an area near a client's genitals, near the coccyx or near a woman's breasts, we need to tell the client in a matter of fact way what we're about to do and why. Let the client decide if it's all right. Watch to see if it really is okay or whether she tenses up or tries to be brave or act cool.

Cautious behavior protects both us and our clients. In the very young and altered state that clients enter into, they can get confused about both our intentions and where our hands actually are. Bring those things into their conscious awareness by giving clients specifics.

We may not know what areas are intrusive for a particular client. Heida Brenneke of the Brenneke School of Massage in Seattle makes a good point, "Massage therapists think too narrowly about where a memory of sexual abuse may be in the body—if, for instance, someone was pinned down by her shoulders, working in that area could bring the memory up." All our work has the potential to trigger a memory of sexual abuse. We therefore want to be alert to clients' responses all the time—tension or other signs of discomfort, such as going numb or leaving their bodies (withdrawing their attention from their bodies.)

Expressing affection: Initiating hugs with clients isn't a good idea. Mandatory hugs can be very intrusive. The same is true, only more so, for kissing on the forehead or cheek. We may think that any expressions of affection would be welcomed by clients. "But love heals—why not hugs?" goes the argument that Lucy Liben of the Swedish Institute in New York hears from some students. Understanding is what heals. And that may involve our understanding that, for some clients, being in charge of their personal space is healing. Let the client initiate hugging.

Unintentional touching: When asked about uncomfortable experiences, clients often cite situations where a practitioner touched them or leaned against them with some part of his body, other than the hands. This is usually accidental on the part of the practitioner, but can be disturbing to the client. A woman reports:

> I was receiving a massage from a male practi-
> tioner and in the middle of it, he leaned against
> my hip with his belly to reach the other side of
> me, instead of walking around the table. I was
> so uncomfortable that I cut the massage short
> and high-tailed it out of there, never to return.

Not every client is going to react that strongly to unintentional or careless touching. However, some will. We want to be respectful of clients' sensitivities. We do not want to prop ourselves against them as if they were furniture. And we want to be careful that we're not wearing sleeves that dangle and things that could brush against clients. In the open and receptive state induced by bodywork, clients shouldn't have to figure out what is touching them.

Erections: Some practitioners routinely discuss with new male clients the possibility that being touched may lead to their having an erection. They might say that although the work itself doesn't have sexual intent, different feelings come and go, arousal being one of them. Erections can be explained as just a normal response to pleasure and being touched, and not a sign of attraction to the practitioner.

Training in School

Several years ago, I asked a group of women Rolfers how they deal with working on the muscle attachments at the top of the pubic bone if the client's penis is in the way. Although these were experienced Rolfers and sophisticated women, their answers involved much giggling and no real solutions, which was partly because we were in a casual social atmosphere and not a classroom. But it was also because the specific issue hadn't been discussed in our training and we were evidently still nervous about it.

While we're in school, the more we can talk through potentially embarrassing dilemmas, the better. Even better is to role play the situation: it is more likely to bring up real feelings. Robert King, president of the Chicago School of Massage, told of a student who was ordinarily "self confident and extroverted:"

> The student was role playing a scene in which she was to tell a sexually aggressive client not to touch her. To her surprise, when she began to act out the situation, she was frozen with fear and couldn't respond. She decided to seek

professional counseling so that she could understand her inability to respond verbally. It was valuable for her to find that out before a client confronted her with such a scenario in her practice.

The Power of Touch

We cannot ignore sexual issues when learning to work with our clients. True, we're not offering sex but we're often offering the pleasure of sensuality and the healing power of touch. The manual therapies are intimate and can bring up all of our issues about sexuality as well as all of our clients' issues.

This work can be a blessing for people who are starved for safe and respectful touch. However, we're always skating the edge between the sacred and the profane. It speaks to the goodwill and compassion of our practitioners that we so often succeed in keeping the balance on the side of the sacred.

Sexual Issues: Protecting Ourselves

❊

Chapter Seven

We live in a culture that sexualizes touch. Many are uneducated about the manual therapies and don't understand that we are professionals who work with therapeutic intention. The intimacy of our work leaves us open to misunderstandings and false accusations. When other practitioners abuse ethical standards, our own professional reputations are damaged by association. How do we protect ourselves from potential confusion and harm—both from the public and from within our ranks?

Mistaken Identity

Some sexual situations aren't complex. For a massage therapist, a common nuisance is being mistaken for someone who is selling sex. As uncomfortable and sometimes scary as this can be, it can usually be handled in a straightforward and uncomplicated way. Diplomatically or forcefully, depending on the situation, the practitioner can simply say some version of, "I'm a health care professional; I don't offer sexual services."

Unfortunately, prostitutes still use "massage" as a cover when they advertise. In some newspapers the ads for "Buffy's Exotica" are right next to our legitimate ads. Plus, to protect themselves from being arrested, prostitutes who advertise their services as massage will, at first, tell a new client that their massage is nonsexual. So we can't blame clients for being confused.

When a client misunderstands, we don't need to waste our energy on a fit of righteous indignation. There's no need to take it personally. Here's a great example of how one massage therapist handled an awkward situation. The story was told to me by Lee Phillips, a massage therapist in Levittown, Pennsylvania:

> A man called and made an appointment. He showed up on time and looked around the room, which was clean and airy with a massage table in the middle, anatomy posters on the walls and books in the bookshelf. The massage therapist was dressed in a polo shirt and long pants, as is her usual style. Seeing the man's perplexed expression, she said "This isn't what you were expecting, is it?"
>
> "Er....uh....no," he mumbled.
>
> "I'll get a phone book for you if you'd like. You may use my phone."
>
> "Uh.....thanks"
>
> She gave him the Yellow Pages, open to "Massage-Other" (which happened to be next to "Massage-Therapeutic") and left the room. Shortly, he came out, said "Thank you" and quickly left.

Never a problem. Never a judgment by either of them.

If the client is on the table and the request for other services isn't made in a threatening or disturbing manner, many massage therapists just say, "I'm a health care professional; I don't

ANSWERING THE DREADED PHONE BOOTH CALL

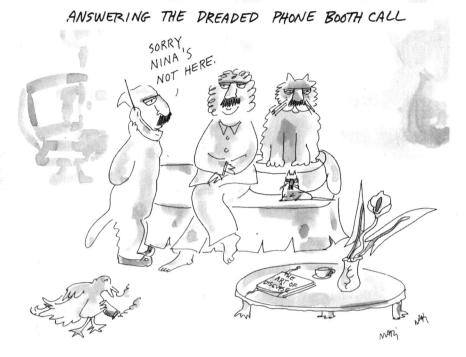

offer sexual services," and that's the end of the discussion. Practitioners tell me that when they have a nonjudgmental, matter-of-fact attitude, clients aren't offended and are able to relax and enjoy the rest of the massage. Massage therapists have different tolerance levels; some wouldn't be comfortable, under any circumstance, working with a person who had made such a request. Ways to handle requests that are threatening or to avoid the situation entirely are discussed below.

The Dreaded Phone Booth Call

When I was a massage therapist in Denver and advertised in the local alternative weekly newspaper, I found it easy to spot the fellows who weren't legitimate: they called from a phone booth. (I could hear the traffic in the background.) They never gave their whole names. They often called on Friday afternoon and they always wanted a massage that day, usually immediately. If someone called and I could hear the traffic sounds, when he asked for Nina, I'd just say, "Sorry, Nina's not here." (Maybe there is some legitimate reason for a client to call from a phone booth, but I wasn't willing to take that chance.)

The client expecting sexual services is more of a problem for massage therapists than other manual therapists. However, even practitioners who don't advertise as massage therapists will occasionally get calls from clients who are confused about what "bodywork" is. People can misunderstand our ads if they are unfamiliar with the kind of work we do. Here are some hints about screening out "massage parlor" clients:

- If you're self-employed and work alone in an office or out of your home, select your clients carefully. Many massage therapists, male and female, who work out of their homes never see a client who wasn't referred by another client or friend.

- Use voice mail rather than your home phone number. If you return calls from your home, be aware that many people have caller I.D. You can block your home phone number when calling a prospective client you don't know.

- When you advertise, avoid the words "release," "total relaxation" and "full body massage." They can sound like veiled sexual references.

- If someone objects to giving you his name and/or phone number, don't see him.

- Ask what types of massage the caller has previously experienced to see if he's ever had a legitimate therapeutic massage or has been to someone you know is a legitimate manual therapist.

- Use your common sense. Don't work in an isolated office with clients you don't know. Don't schedule new clients late in the day or at times when no one else is around.

- An office setting is safer and more professional than your home. Leading a client through your home to where the bedrooms are (and your office now is) can be suggestive to both male and female clients and frightening to some.

- Trust your intuition. If you get an uncomfortable feeling, pay attention. If you feel uneasy during the initial phone call, don't make the appointment.

- Practitioners need to be especially careful about outcalls. Outcalls put you in the most danger. You're going into someone else's home and what happens can get out of your control. You're at the mercy of any hidden agendas the client might have.

> One male massage therapist related a story of being set-up by a female client who wanted to make her boyfriend jealous. During the outcall, the client threw the draping off her chest just as her boyfriend burst through the door. The boyfriend made angry accusations; the massage therapist fled, unharmed but wiser.

Screen your outcalls carefully or only do outcalls with people who've been referred by someone you trust.

Refusing To Work With A Client

We can refuse to work with a client at any time from the first phone call to the end of the session. We don't have to work with a client who is rude or coarse or who won't take "no" for an answer. We don't have to finish a massage.

If a practitioner wishes to end a session in progress, she or he can say, "I'm not comfortable working with you anymore," or "I'm sorry—perhaps you don't mean anything by what you're saying, but I'm just not comfortable working with you anymore." If we were to say, "You're acting like a creep," the client could engage us in an argument about whether or not he is indeed acting like a creep. If we just talk about what we feel, there's no arguing with that.

Once the session is terminated, the practitioner can tell the client that she'll wait outside while he gets dressed. Most massage therapists are so grateful to get rid of such clients that they don't ask for payment. (Others get payment at the start of a session.) Technically he may owe the fee for a massage or half a massage, but if there's a chance of violence, don't make an issue of it. We don't want to put ourselves at risk.

Some massage clinics post signs stating that they reserve the right to terminate a session based on issues of sexual innuendo or conduct. Some massage therapists ask new clients to sign an agreement to that effect on their history/intake form. The more we can make it clear from the beginning that we do a therapeutic massage and this is a non-sexual situation, the easier it is.

Self-Presentation

If we are getting a high percentage of calls or office encounters in which the clients think we're offering sex, we need to take a look at how we're presenting ourselves. This could be as simple as changing our ads or how we dress or as complicated as looking at what our intentions really are. In any case, we need to get another perspective—we could ask a mentor or more experienced practitioner for help.

Predatory Behavior

There are people in every profession who use their roles to take advantage of clients sexually, and ours is no exception. I don't mean well-intentioned practitioners who have stumbled into a destructive situation or made a mistake in judgment; I mean someone who frequently seduces clients or violates their sexual boundaries, someone who is indifferent to the emotional damage he causes.

Because of the power difference between practitioner and client, and all the ways that clients on the table are vulnerable to us, the practitioner violating a client's sexual boundaries can cause trauma. The example below was in *Massage Therapy Journal*:

> A female spa client felt inappropriately touched by a male massage therapist and filed a lawsuit. The therapist, who it turned out had a history of complaints against him by female clients, had worked with her with no draping and with her knees up, genitals exposed. As he worked, he ran his fingers down her adductors close to her genitals, within an inch. She froze and didn't say anything at the time, letting him finish the massage.

In the weeks after this incident, she became increasingly depressed and so anxious that it was difficult for her to go to work. She began having nightmares and gained 35 pounds. She grew fearful of traveling alone or being in enclosed rooms. Finally, she went to a doctor, who diagnosed her with post-traumatic stress syndrome. (We don't know whether the client had previous abuse but it sounds probable.) Tracing her sudden downhill spiral back to the massage, she contacted a lawyer and decided to sue.

The legal part ended with an out-of-court settlement. We don't know how the client fared emotionally, how long it took for her to come out of her depression and state of anxiety, or if she ever did.

Over the years, our profession has reflected the culture in its increasing sensitivity to sexual harassment and misuse of power. In the late seventies and early eighties, there wasn't the awareness of the ways that dating a client or flirting with a student were unethical. However, as a profession, we have become increasingly aware of the damage that can be done by crossing boundaries.

We have also reflected the culture in coming to an understanding that seductiveness isn't about sex and affection; it's about dominance and hostility. The practitioner involved in *habitual* predatory behavior often is a sociopath, that is, a seductive charmer who has no concern about the harm done to his/her victims. Habitual predators do great harm to clients and to the reputation of the profession. It's in the interest of the profession to find ways to expose them and shut them down.

No Witch Hunts

I'm not advocating witch hunts. In contemporary culture, people have become too quick to point the finger, jump into lawsuits or drag people's names through the mud for little or no reason. There's no healing in such actions.

We want to be very careful about false accusations. Spreading rumors and unsubstantiated gossip can harm the reputation of an innocent person, affecting her/his livelihood. Aside from being unkind and unethical, it can subject us to slander suits from the accused.

When we have reason to question another practitioner's ethics, the decent way to handle it is to approach the practitioner directly in a manner that shows we're looking for information and haven't yet drawn conclusions. The first step is to have the courage to make a phone call to the person or to write a letter: "I've heard this about you. I thought you needed to know what is being said so that you can respond to it."

If the accusations prove to be true, we want to distinguish the unrepentant and habitual offender from the momentarily confused and off-balance practitioner. Ethics procedures need to be written and implemented in a way that stops the predators and helps the others. We want to create an atmosphere within which practitioners can feel safe talking about their confusion without a misstep getting blown out of proportion. At the same time, we need clarity about what constitutes unethical practice and what harm such behavior does to clients.

A practitioner who is advised that his or her behavior is unethical should give assurance that the behavior will stop immediately, assuming that the rumors are found to be true. If confrontation doesn't lead to a change in behavior, then we need to go through the appropriate channels of whatever professional association or licensing board is relevant. In that way, confidentiality is (or should be) guaranteed.

Dealing with Predatory Behavior

Predators are a problem across the board—they crop up in all different kinds of manual therapy, regardless of how incompatible their behavior is with the underlying philosophy of their training. Predators give the manual therapies a bad name; they damage the reputation of the other practitioners who work near them, especially those who do their brand of work.

I've talked with practitioners all over the country who have tried to stop predators in their bodywork communities and their cities, and the dynamics are very similar— it's usually a difficult process. As happens with other professionals, such suits usually involve female clients and male practitioners. Female clients who have been harassed or mistreated sometimes feel that they colluded with the predator and are ashamed to take action. Also, women who are taken in by a predator are frequently women who are not emotionally strong and may not make good witnesses—they can be dismissed as "hysterical" or "flaky." The accusers themselves, the actual victims or those acting on behalf of the victims, can become the target of either hostility or legal action from the accused and from his supporters. This is particularly true if the accuser and the predator are in the same bodywork community. Sides can be taken and the situation can become divisive.

Even if the accuser isn't under attack himself, taking someone to court or filing a complaint is time-consuming and emotionally wrenching. Incidents have to be carefully documented, victims have to be persuaded to participate, legal advice has to be obtained. The task is difficult. It takes time and energy away from work and personal life, and it requires a good deal of support from colleagues. However, those pursuing such a complaint are performing a service both for the profession and for future would-be victims of that practitioner.

Protecting Ourselves from Complaints and Lawsuits

As discussed in the previous chapter, any practitioner can be complained about by any client. However, those who are in a group that is generally perceived as sexually aggressive, whether or not that perception is accurate, are more likely to be complained about or sued. Since most complaints are by female clients against male practitioners, men, as a whole, are more at risk. In conservative parts of the country, minority men can be even more at risk, as well as homosexual practitioners. All of us who touch people need to be cautious about sexual boundaries, but practitioners in those groups should take extra precautions. The next sections will discuss ways to become more aware.

Avoiding lawsuits is also discussed in Chapter Five on Ethics.

Fatal Attractions: The Unbalanced and Seductive Client
There are instances of unbalanced and seductive clients causing problems for male bodyworkers. (All of the instances I've
heard involve female clients and male practitioners, but the
situation could be a male client and a female practitioner or
same sex client and practitioner.)

> A male massage school teacher was seduced by
> a female client, who had, a few months earlier,
> been a student in a class where he had assisted.
> As is often the case with unbalanced people,
> she had "an exquisite sense" of how to connect
> with him and make him feel special. She made
> him feel that making love to her was a heroic
> and generous act.
>
> She then turned on him and enlisted another
> student to get him in trouble with the school.
> The woman had a history of childhood sexual
> abuse and though she had been the aggressor
> and a willing participant, she began to experi-
> ence their sexual relationship as though she had
> been an unwilling victim. The teacher ended
> up with a damaged reputation.

Even without inappropriate behavior, the practitioner can be
falsely accused.

> Another male bodyworker described narrowly
> escaping disaster when an emotionally dis-
> turbed client pleaded with him to have sex with
> her. She gave him assurances that she wasn't
> the type to get attached. When he still refused,

she set about trying to harm him. She went to
the police to check the legalities of his license;
she called his landlord and reported he was
having wild orgies. None of these actions caused
him permanent damage, but he was glad that
he had not gone along with the seduction.

How do we guard against such clients? What are the warning
signs? As discussed in Chapter Five on Ethics, there are the red
flags of "specialness" and of "rescuing." Some mentally unbalanced clients are experts at making us feel special. They know
just the right buttons to push. The bodyworker who related
both stories (and was himself the practitioner in the second
story) reported, "Both the other male practitioner and I felt
that we were nobly responding to the true needs of the client.
I thought of my client, for example, as an extraordinarily sensitive being who only needed support and recognition to realize her full potential. The other bodyworker felt like a knight
on a white horse saving the fair maiden."

When we feel like noble rescuers, we are probably responding
to some deep wish in the client that comes from the client's
early childhood. This kind of intense transference is highly
volatile and can quickly change to disappointment and rage.

We need to be alert to the signs of emotional seduction. Does
this client make us feel unusually attractive, competent or sensitive? Do we think of him/her as being special? The countertransference in these cases can feel as if a spell has been cast.
We can break the spell by getting a good dose of reality from a
grounded professional that we trust. And we can remember
that there's never a good reason to have sex with a client or
student.

The Nice Guy Blind Spot

Many of us don't understand transference—however, the danger is greater for the male practitioner who doesn't. If he doesn't fully realize the power of a woman's unconscious attitudes about men and the possible memories of sexual abuse that she may bring to the table, he can be stepping into trouble. Some men apparently think that because they are "nice guys" or happily married, female clients will somehow be able to automatically feel comfortable with them. Charles Wiltsie, a massage therapist who conducts ethics classes for men, says that men may not understand how frightening the possibility of inappropriate touch and speech is to many women. He says that they don't sufficiently understand that for women clients, "The smallest error or slip of a hand can change a relaxing experience into a nightmare."[*]

Another problem is that the take-charge behavior that works for men in many situations may not serve them as manual therapists. Here's an example:

> A male massage therapy student was partnered with a female student to learn the techniques for back work. When he began working, he unsnapped her bra without asking her. A teacher noticed what he'd done and the startled reaction of the female student. When the male student was asked to explain his actions, he said, "I thought it would be easier for me to get to her back muscles without the bra in the way."

It's understandable for a student to be focused on learning technique, but goal-oriented behavior isn't necessarily helpful

---

[*]Charles W. Wiltsie III, "Uniquely Male: Ethics in Massage Therapy," *Massage and Bodywork*, April/May 1999, 46.)

in manual therapists. As practitioners, men will be safer from misunderstandings if they let the client run the show. Clients need to know they are in charge of what happens, especially when the gender dynamics are male practitioner/female client.

Ultimately, the underlying beliefs and sensitivity of the practitioner are what will come through to the client. Education and dialogue are the cure for blind spots—the way to become attuned to transference issues that can alter a woman's perception in ways that put male practitioners at risk.

The Importance of Dialogue and Education

William Greenberg, the Grievance Chairman for the American Massage Therapy Association, notes there's been a recent drop in sexual harassment complaints. Greenberg attributes this to the fact that schools are giving more instruction in what constitutes sexual harassment and boundary violations.

Charles Wiltsie believes that male manual therapists may need a men-only forum in which to discuss ethics problems. He thinks that men are often outnumbered in classes, especially men who are massage therapists, and may not feel free to talk about their experiences with women present.

There's no doubt that more honest dialogue would help, whether it's male to male or male to female and whether it's in school or in post-graduate classes. Manual therapists need more honest dialogue with each other—to listen with interest and respect to the other gender's concerns. Male practitioners rightfully fear false accusation that could damage their careers. Women practitioners understandably have more knowledge about the fears that female clients bring to a session.

Confusion and Imperfection

Manual therapists have to make an extra effort to combat the public misconception that links our work with sexual services. How often have we seen massage therapists portrayed in television sitcoms or movies as crossing the line? How often have new acquaintances made sexual innuendoes and "jokes" about our work?

Because of those misconceptions, we can sometimes go too far in the other direction and expect ourselves, as professionals, never to have sexual thoughts about our clients or to make mistakes about sexual boundaries. We can be reluctant to talk honestly with each other. We may not want to expose our imperfection and confusion. A school administrator said that faculty in her school were reluctant to teach classes in sexual ethics for that reason. Because they didn't think they had achieved perfection in their own sexual attitudes or behavior, they didn't feel qualified to set themselves up as "experts."

The sexual issues related to our work are dangerous ones for manual therapists, as individual practitioners and as a profession. Misunderstandings, inappropriate behavior and accusations related to sex are the most damaging to both practitioner and to the profession. How do we lower the risk and keep our work environment safe for ourselves and therapeutic for our clients? We need to do our own personal work about sexual issues, whether in supervision or counseling. We need to have more honest discussion among fellow students and colleagues. And we need to soften our attitudes so that we can allow for imperfection and confusion in ourselves and others, while at the same time, stop the behaviors that harm clients.

Getting Comfortable with Money

�֍

Chapter Eight

Many of us have an uneasy relationship with business finances. We feel awkward going from being the Caring One when a client is on the table, to being the Cashier at the end of the session who says, "Now gimme sixty bucks." We feel a little guilty about money.

A bodyworker said recently, "I'm not in this for the money. This work is like a calling for me." For those with that attitude, there's often an accompanying anti-money sentiment. There's nothing wrong with wanting to make the world better, but there's no need to feel awkward or guilty about money either. Part of what professional means, after all, is that this is how we pay the rent. Charging appropriate fees tells a client that we're serious about our work.

Massage school directors report that students generally have a hard time charging for their work. New practitioners feel uncomfortable because they think they're charging people for nurturing them or caring about them. A colleague has this advice: "Tell them that clients are paying for their time. The caring is free."

The Case for Money

Actually, the exchange of money is part of what makes clients feel safe. Money clarifies clients' obligations to us and ours to them. The exchange of money helps clients feel comfortable

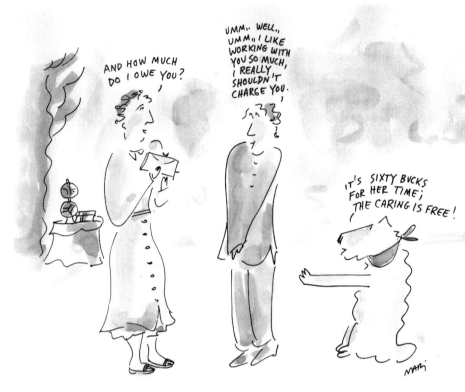

with receiving what we give them. They know what they owe us in return. Money's clean, it's precise, it's simple. It balances the relationship.

Paying for services is an important part of the client's healing process, not an unpleasant bit of reality that we tack onto the "real" healing process. Throughout the world, fees are an intrinsic aspect of healing. Jerome Frank studied many kinds of health care providers—witch doctors, traditional Western medical doctors and alternative health practitioners. In *Persuasion and Healing*, he describes the ways that an effective therapeutic experience involves the patient/client making a sacrifice. In cultures other than our own, the sacrifice might be a nice fat chicken. In ours, it's usually money.

The idea of the healing value of sacrifice doesn't justify greed or over-charging, but the concept can help us feel more comfortable with collecting appropriate fees. The element of sacrifice may give clients a deeper sense of the treatment's value and help them benefit from it. Many manual therapists have discovered that clients who are given a "special deal" or who are undercharged never seem to get as much out of the work as those who pay full price.

The exchange of money provides clarity; it's part of a safe professional environment. It validates both practitioner and client. The giving and receiving of money speaks deeply to us about our worth and the value of our work. For clients, it's a tangible sign of how much they will invest in their own well-being.

Different Modes

The part of us that empathizes with clients and the part of us that makes budgets and deals with money are two different aspects of our personalities. Sometimes it can feel awkward to make a transition between the two. Doctors and people who do volume business resolve the conflict by having another person, an office manager, handle the finances. But most of us are stuck with the dilemma of sliding back and forth between Caring One and Cashier.

> We've just finished a session in which we felt touched by a client's revelation of the pain he feels in his life, and we're feeling compassionate toward him. As he gets ready to pay, he says, "Oh, do you mind if I postdate this check

for next week?" Or, "Gee, I forgot my check-
book. Mind if I pay you next time?" How do
we then say, "I prefer that you pay me at the
end of each session," without feeling callous?
Much easier to say "Oh, sure...that's fine," even
if it really isn't fine.

The majority of us don't come to this work with a business
background. We spend much of our time in school learning
our trade, not learning how to sell ourselves and collect our
fees. To move past any blocks we might have, we have to put
extra energy into educating ourselves through mentors, classes
and supervision.

Money and Sex

Money is like sex—we talk about it all the time but rarely do
we talk about it honestly or openly. When openness is lacking,
we don't realize that others are struggling with the same issues.
We don't learn from each other's mistakes and we can't support each other.

Is there a practitioner who has had perfect judgment about the
financial part of the business... and do we even know what
"perfect" would look like? Is there anyone who hasn't backed
down from charging a client for an appointment canceled at
the last minute, who hasn't given a special discount that back-
fired or who hasn't ever under or overcharged?

Money is also like sex in that it brings up strong feelings. Many
of us have old, unexamined ideas that get in the way of our
judgment. We might have deep feelings about whether money
is "good" or "bad," or whether we are competent with it. We

might have unrealistic ideas about how hard or easy it is to make a living. Also, we have to come to terms with cultural values that measure personal worth by one's bank account. Working in a profession that usually doesn't make us rich, we have to learn to value our work even if we probably won't become millionaires (or even close).

Money is also like sex in that we can lose clients very quickly if they misunderstand our intentions or we become careless about boundaries. For instance, suddenly changing fees without notice can be jolting to a client, as can charging for a missed appointment without having explained our policy at the outset.

Because we have strong feelings about money, there's all the more reason to talk about it—with a mentor or with a support group of peers. And all the more reason to be clear with ourselves and our clients about financial policies. Because we can be swayed by strong feelings, we want to stick with our policies unless we have a carefully thought-out reason to make an exception.

What to Charge?

Starting a practice, most of us can judge what the going rate is for our brand of manual therapy at our level of experience by researching the fees other manual therapists charge. All the same, we still want to give careful thought to what we charge. Our rates affect what both clients and colleagues will think about us.

If we charge more than the norm, some clients may be put off, while others may think we must be offering something special to be charging extra. If we charge less than the going rate, some may be attracted to the bargain, but they may not value the work as much.

If we charge a good deal (maybe $20) over or under what others are charging, we run the risk of alienating our colleagues. Sometimes even $10 a session over or under can set a practitioner apart. Colleagues may feel we're arrogant if we charge more than they do without having more training or experience. They may feel we are undercutting them if we charge less than the usual fee. Mostly, we want to settle on an amount with which we feel comfortable. If we're not comfortable, people will sense it.

Talking To Clients About Money

When we talk with clients about our money policies, our attitude and tone make a world of difference. We want to sound straightforward, business-like and confident—not either apologetic or punitive. For instance, if we have to let clients know that we are charging them for a missed appointment, we can simply say, "As you know, I charge full fee for a missed appointment." Of course, we want to make sure they know from the beginning what our policies are.

Clients want to go to practitioners who are confident. If we are giving notice that we will be raising our fees, for instance, we don't need to sound apologetic. As a colleague said, "We don't need to send clients a sympathy card when we raise our fees." Tone makes all the difference.

The Perils of the Special Deal

What about giving discounts or using sliding scales? Most of the people I interviewed found it works best to stick with one fee—with rare and well-thought-out exceptions.

The money arena is one in which we're likely to feel tempted to make special exceptions for clients. Making exceptions occasionally works out and is appropriate; most of the time, it's a mistake and a sign of deeper problems. We want to treat each client as a unique person, but we can run into trouble when we start bending money boundaries.

When we give a discount or use a sliding scale, we're automatically creating a dual relationship. We become the client's banker—involving ourselves in his finances. As practitioners, we shouldn't be concerned with how much or how little money a client has. Dual relationships create complications that can interfere with our ability to put our heart into our work. Imagine this scenario:

> A client has convinced you that, as a student, she can't afford your full fee. You have agreed to accept $40 per session instead of your usual $60 fee. After you've seen her for a month or two, she tells you she can't make the next week's regular appointment because she's taking a vacation to Hawaii. How do you feel?

> Or same client comes in after a month or two and complains that she's not getting enough from the work, that she doesn't feel as good as she wants to. Are you able to handle this complaint with the same objectivity that you would if she were a full-fee client? Or do you judge her as ungrateful?

Sometimes schools or individuals give discounts to groups of people, such as students, people with life-threatening illnesses, or spiritual/religious teachers and ministers. A special fee can work well if it's motivated by our hearts or our convictions and not by guilt. When we make such an exception, we need to keep checking in to make sure our hearts are still in it and our bank balances aren't suffering.

Even when we do pro bono (no fee) work or discounted work that seems purely altruistic, we want to look at the difficulties that may be hidden in such relationships. Good questions to ask ourselves any time we consider reducing fees are:

- Do we have a standard policy for fee reduction and are we veering from that policy?
- Are we uncomfortable with saying "no" to this client?
- How do we decide how much discount to give?
- Is there any way we foresee coming to resent or regret the arrangement or wish it were different? Will we feel owed?
- What are the possibilities the special arrangement will harm the therapeutic relationship?

By not carelessly making special deals, we protect both ourselves and our clients. The special financial arrangements we make for clients often don't help them. When we go outside the usual fee structure, it can confuse clients: they can end up feeling uncertain what their obligation to us is. They also may wonder if we can adequately provide a safe, consistent environment or if we will continue to change the boundaries.

When a session is free or at a reduced rate, we need to be especially careful with other boundaries. It would be confusing to a reduced fee client, for instance, to also allow him to come in twenty minutes late for a session. (It would be confusing to anyone but especially for someone for whom we are already bending boundaries in other ways.) Such allowances can also create resentment in us.

Sometimes there's a bit of an unhealthy "rescue" attitude in a special deal. In an unhealthy "rescue," we, usually unconsciously, treat the client as if he were in some way inadequate and therefore, not able to be held to normal business arrangements. Sometimes, clients attempt to manipulate us into such thinking. Sometimes, we may think giving a client a special deal shows our compassion. All of these motivations are different from making an adult-to-adult business arrangement with someone who has a legitimate reason to need a discount. As noted in Chapter Five on Ethics, unhealthy rescues always backfire. When we depart from our normal framework, we encourage clients to do so. A colleague reports:

> After I made a special payment arrangement for a client who said he was down on his luck, he missed two appointments without giving me notice. After we were finished with our work, I had a hard time collecting what he owed me.

It would be difficult to make blanket statements about when it is appropriate to give a discount. Some practitioners can handle giving discounts and making special arrangements more easily than others. We have to know our own limitations and biases about money. The bottom line is whether the arrangement could be harmful to either us or the client.

Missed Appointments

You've arranged your life to see a new client at 3 p.m. You're not at the movie, you're not taking a nap, you're not hanging out with your buddies. You have kept that slot open for that client and you're all prepared: you've warmed up the room, put clean sheets on the table. Maybe you were counting on the money and you've already mentally spent the fifty dollars. And what happens? No show. No phone messages to explain.... nothing. The missed appointment is that dreadful thud in the professional life of a manual therapist.

Along with the dreadful thud goes the pesky question of whether to ask the client to pay for the missed session. Most manual therapists usually charge for a missed appointment unless there's been an emergency. But what constitutes an authentic emergency is a judgment call. Illness rarely comes on suddenly. Cars don't often just stop working. Traffic is usually predictable. Sometimes no-show clients can't anticipate problems, but often they can.

Many of the manual therapists I interviewed were flexible about missed appointments; for instance, some don't charge the first time a client misses. However, standard practice is to charge full or partial fee for a no-show. Some practitioners—especially new ones—find it hard to ask a client to pay for a missed appointment. They feel awkward asking payment for "doing nothing." The point is that the practitioner could have booked another client in that slot. It's time and money lost.

If the no-show client doesn't call to explain or to make another appointment and won't return our calls, obviously we can't do anything about it. Such a client probably wouldn't respond to a written bill either. Sometimes practitioners are concerned about making the client angry, so they rationalize that they wouldn't have filled the vacancy anyway. Nevertheless, do we really want to work with a client who doesn't respect our time? If we feel angry with a client for missing appointments without notice, can we be compassionate when we work with her?

Sticking to our guns about charging for missed appointments shows that we value our time as professionals. In this instance, maintaining boundaries protects *us* and helps *us* feel safe. The flip side is that we show clients the same courtesy, letting them know that if we have to cancel their appointments without 24 hour's notice, they will receive a free or discounted session.

Even with a firm policy that has been communicated to clients, we will always have an occasional no-show. I've had no-shows from clients who have heard my policy twice as part of a standard orientation and who have also signed a written agreement. Here are some suggestions to make missed appointments less frequent:

- When clients make their first appointments, always tell them that they will be charged for appointments canceled without 24 hours (or whatever we think is adequate) cancellation notice.

- Have clients sign an agreement to that effect the first time we see them. Even if we are sure we have told them, they may not remember that we did.

- Tell unreliable clients that they need to call us by a certain time the day before the session to confirm the appointment or we will fill that time slot with someone else.

Refunds

It's often wise to offer an unhappy client a refund or partial refund even if there has been no negligence or harm on the part of the practitioner. If a client is upset enough to want fees refunded, we're generally better off giving the money back. Practitioners may want to consult a lawyer about how best to handle a specific situation.

If a client is harmed or neglected during our work with him—whether or not we were totally responsible—then we want to make it up to the client.

> A woman had received four sessions from a bodyworker. The fifth one was 20 minutes shorter than the others and the quality of the work seemed below the previous quality. After leaving his office, she realized she felt short-changed and called the bodyworker, explaining what she had noticed. He told her that she was right—that he had been on the verge of catching the flu when he worked with her. He didn't apologize or offer a refund or discount on another session. The client never went back to him and didn't refer anyone else to him.

This example doesn't mean that whenever we feel we have performed less than our best, we should rush to offer a free session. Those who are self-critical would be constantly offering free sessions. It does mean that when a client feels short-changed and has reason to feel that way, we want to make it up to him. Regardless of whether we had control over the situation that caused a client's discomfort, not charging full fee or refunding our fee is the smart thing to do if we want to continue seeing the client. An example of this is a massage therapist who charged a client for only half a session when the last 10 minutes of the hour were disrupted by the loud barking of the neighbor's dog. (Although we may not be able to control the neighbor's dog, it's our responsibility to provide a quiet environment for the session.)

Advertising

Manual therapists are essentially running a small business and small businesses advertise. Many of us don't have previous experience in business or as entrepreneurs. We may be uncomfortable with basic business practices and feel that the idea of advertising or promoting ourselves is distasteful. Some of us have been taught that we're not supposed to "toot our own horns." But there's a difference between inflated bragging and honestly telling people the benefits of our work.

We can change our view of advertising by thinking of it as education: letting prospective clients know what's available and how it might help them. No need to feel like used car salesmen—when we educate the public about our work, we are teachers.

Help with Money Awareness

To become comfortable with running a small business, we need a better understanding of our own attitudes about money. Reading a book or hearing rules or suggestions about money isn't usually enough help. Some massage school business classes use role playing in various situations as a way to unearth our real feelings about money. For instance, role-playing telling a reluctant client that he owes for canceling without enough notice would be useful. Also, having mentors who are clean in their relationship to money can be a major help with business issues. Peer group discussions can be supportive because everyone has money and practice issues, but generally in different areas. In a group, others will have clarity about issues that we struggle with. Personal supervision can also aid us in getting to the deeper issues that we have about money.

Some manual therapists are starting to use "coaches"—individuals specifically trained to help practitioners create business goals that suit their values. A coach can help us figure out the steps to reach those goals and then, like a personal exercise trainer, hold us accountable each week for making progress.

There are also workshops that specialize in getting to the bottom of our attitudes about money. To find a good workshop or coach, we can look for a well-recommended one that has made a beneficial change in the financial attitudes of someone we know.

Getting More Comfortable with Money

Both personally and as a group, manual therapists' issues about money are sometimes rooted in insecurity about our professional worth. Most of us don't have backgrounds as "captains of industry"—in fact, many of us are suspicious of anything that smacks of big business. We can be naive or mistrustful about money.

Our work isn't an easy way to make a living and we need all the help we can get. By exchanging ideas with colleagues, mentors and people who have been successful in business, we can educate ourselves and find what works for us. As we become more conscious about our relationship to money, the financial aspect of our work can be more satisfying.

The ability to set good money boundaries is a crucial part of our work. Clients need the comfort and safety of a clear financial relationship, and so do we. Keeping clean and clear about money is, like most boundary issues, a skill and an art that we will practice and improve throughout our careers.

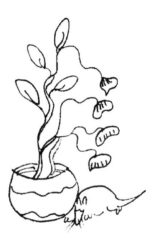

Dual Relationships: Wearing Many Hats

✤

Chapter Nine

Dual relationships—having more than one relationship with a client—are practically a tradition in our profession. We almost think we have a right to them. We can become indignant about the idea that we might want to limit or even eliminate these relationships: "What! I can't have coffee with a client?" "My buddy Bob has been coming to me for years and it's just fine." "Where would I get clients if not from people I know?"

It's true that we can stretch the boundaries more than, for instance, psychotherapists can. Beginning psychotherapists can't practice counseling with those close to them, but massage therapy students can try out their strokes on friends and relatives. Sometimes it works for manual therapists to see friends as clients or to do trades or to see a student as a client. For the most part, however, dual relationships cause problems—they create stress in our practices and short-change our clients.

> A massage therapist told me that she had begun a trade with an old friend—she would give him massages and he would paint her living room. He wasn't a professional painter, but she thought he could do a good job. Because there were too many possible confusions and misunderstandings in both working with friends *and* doing trades, I advised her not to go through with it. Despite these objections, the

massage therapist continued with the trade. She thought the problems would be small and she said she really needed to have her living room painted and didn't want to pay a professional.

Knowing my interest in dual relationships, she was conscientious enough to call a few weeks later and report how unsatisfactory the trade had been. She herself hadn't been satisfied with her behavior during the sessions—she found herself talking about mutual friends or her own concerns. She thought it may have felt more like a social visit than a session to her friend as well, since he often treated their appointments with the casualness of a social visit—sometimes showing up late or making several phone calls before getting on the table. Because he was a friend, she had a hard time asserting herself and asking him to be on time and ready.

After she had finished her part of the trade, he painted the living room, but she felt the quality of the work was poor. When she tried to discuss her dissatisfaction with him, he became defensive. With some reluctance, he did re-do some of the work. She ended up feeling short-changed, he felt offended and their friendship suffered.

It's difficult, for many reasons, for even experienced practitioners to work with friends. Often both parties are tempted to treat sessions as social, rather than professional, occasions—

being careless about time, for instance, or not keeping the focus on the client. Ongoing trades, especially of bodywork, can be difficult to keep balanced in terms of each person feeling that the arrangement is fair. There is also the emotional confusion of switching back and forth from client to practitioner, from taker to giver.

Transference and Dual Relationships

Dual relationships rarely take into account the power of transference. In the story above, the painter may have become accustomed to seeing his friend as the nurturer because of her role as his massage therapist. This could have made it hard for him to appropriately become attentive to his friend's needs when he was in the role of painter.

Switching roles can lead to all kinds of confusion. It's easy to say or do something that interferes with the therapeutic environment if we have another involvement with the client.

My first Rolfing client was someone I already knew as an acquaintance. While she was going through the basic ten session series, she and I were involved in the same community project.

In the middle of the ten sessions—a time when the client's body and sense of self is changing but has not yet come to resolution, a time when the client is counting on her Rolfer to help her find a more balanced place—my client called about a detail of the community project and also asked me how I was doing. Caught up in deadlines, I breezily said, "Oh, I'm losing my mind."

Later when we were talking about how the Rolfing process had gone for her, she told me how much that had upset her. "Do you know what it's like to have your Rolfer tell you she's losing her mind?" My casual remark would have been appropriate with a colleague, but not with a client.

Dual Relationships: Ease and Scarcity

Why are dual relationships often so compelling? Like the massage therapist in the first story who was trading to have her living room painted, why do we sometimes plunge ahead with them, even though we know the potential problems? A colleague reports:

> I never socialize with my clients or even ex-clients, so I was surprised to find myself thinking about asking my ex-client Mary to attend a concert with me. I realized that I was drawn to this unusual boundary-bending because I was lonely. A good friend had recently moved away, and I had a gap in my social life. I felt tempted to fill it with an ex-client I really liked and who I knew liked me. Once I realized what the problem was, I began thinking of other ways to find new friends.

A practitioner needs a friend. A bodyworker needs to have her living room painted. A new massage therapist needs clients and her friends are the only people who know she's ready for business. One of the reasons we initiate dual relationships is that they seem so easy and convenient. We don't have to find another way to find a friend or pay a professional to paint the room or advertise in the larger community. Trades can feel like we're getting something almost for free (even though the IRS expects us to report trades as income). However, as in the story of the massage therapist and the friend/painter, dual relationships usually create more trouble than they're worth. What may seem easy at first can later become bogged down by misunderstandings.

Fear may be another reason we can have a hard time giving up dual relationships—fear of not having enough clients or friends or money to pay someone else. Perhaps fear is also what fuels practitioners' strong objections to limiting their dual relationships. When we take on a friend as a client because we really "need" the money or we do a trade because we "can't afford" to get massage any other way or we make friends with a client because we "don't know anyone else," we're acting out of fear. However, decisions to work with a client need to be made using objective professional standards, not out of a fear of scarcity in our lives.

Minimizing the Problems

Often it's hard to avoid dual relationships. Sometimes we have good reason to take on a friend as a client or do a trade or even socialize with an ex-client. We may be the only St. John's Neuromuscular or cranial-sacral or Aston Patterning practitioner in town, and our friend would benefit from that method. We may be the only massage therapist that a shy friend would be comfortable seeing. We may be part of a community in which it's hard to avoid social contact between clients and practitioners. When do dual relationships work and when do they harm both participants? How can we manage dual relationships gracefully, with the least stress to the client and ourselves?

Cautions

First, here are situations in which we would *not* want to make an exception—situations where a dual relationship could be harmful. They might work as a one-time session but not as an ongoing therapeutic relationship:

- Practitioners of emotionally-oriented or psychologically-oriented body work should avoid dual relationships. Those practitioners are always working with deep transference issues and can't risk the confusion that would arise.

- It's best not to work with friends who are actively dealing with abuse issues or in crisis. The likelihood of intense transference and/or dependency in those situations makes it difficult to work well with someone we know socially.

- Sexual relationships with clients are forbidden and with ex-clients are limited.

- Involving clients or ex-clients in another business relationship verges on the unethical. (See Chapter Five on ethical decisions.)

Converting clients to friends, business associates or lovers is more problematic than the other way around. Because of transference, we run into more ethical problems when we try to make a client into a friend or some other kind of relationship than when we turn a friend, acquaintance or business associate into a client. Clients and former clients deserve careful handling during even casual social encounters, since we may still be disproportionately important to them.

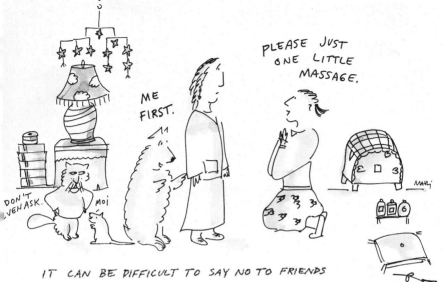

IT CAN BE DIFFICULT TO SAY NO TO FRIENDS
WHO WANT "FREE SAMPLES".

Avoid Mixing Social Occasions with Work

Just as we don't want sessions to be about socializing, social gatherings aren't an appropriate place to display our professional talents. Even when we're students and not charging, if someone asks us to rub a sore shoulder and we're outside our offices or work space, it's not a good idea. It can be difficult to turn down friends who want free samples, but we can just smile and say, "I'm off duty" or " Why don't we set up a time for you to come see me in my therapy room?" People need to know that it's unfair to ask us to be available all the time. Also, we can tell them that we can do a better job when we have the appropriate environment and our attention can be focused solely on them.

The same is true for consulting at a party about someone's sore back. It's tempting to want to show off or sell our work in a social gathering, but we can't really give someone our full attention at a party. It's not an appropriate setting for a professional consultation. We can give out our business card and ask the person to call during business hours. We can say, "I'd really like to discuss it with you, but I can't really do you justice in an atmosphere like this. Why don't you call me Monday and I'll be glad to talk with you more."

Working with Friends and Relatives

In general, this isn't a good idea. Some practitioners never work with friends or relatives because of boundary considerations. Professionals need to work with an objective, nonjudgmental attitude and not have their own agendas for a client. Clients need to be able to focus on themselves and not be aware of our needs. Those goals are just about impossible when we work with people who are involved in our lives in other ways.

If friends want sessions, it's best to let them know that they would probably benefit more from going to a practitioner they don't know. Friends rarely give us the authority we deserve or take the work as seriously as they would with someone they don't know, which takes away from their sessions.

Occasionally we can make exceptions, but not often. We can sometimes see a friend or family member on a one-time basis or every few months and not have problems, but it's not a good idea to see a friend on an ongoing basis or for a series of sessions. When we do work with friends and family, we can use the following guidelines to make the work safer and easier for both practitioner and client. Practitioners need to be aware of the extra energy it will take for them to keep appropriate boundaries. (Imagine the effort it takes to not chat with a friend during a session.) Dual relationships can add strain to our work day.

Confidentiality: We need to emphasize to our friends and family that what they say and do inside a session will be held in confidence, and also, that we won't talk with them about sessions outside the office space.

Separate social time and professional: Let them know that it works better if we don't mix social and professional time—if we don't chit-chat during a session or go to lunch together right before or after a session. It's a good idea to entirely avoid seeing the friend socially while he/she is a client, or at the very least, we shouldn't take the friendship to another level. If someone is, for instance, a friend that we have lunch with every few months, we don't want to start having lunch every week during our work with them.

Don't relax boundaries and framework standards: Because we're already bending boundaries by working with a friend, we need to be more aware of all other boundaries and framework, not less. We may be tempted to think, "Oh, it's just old Bob...I can be late or still be eating my sandwich when he arrives." That would give Bob a message that the setting is not quite professional or safe for him. Aside from interfering with his ability to relax, it's bad advertising for the practitioner. Every client is a potential source of referrals and if someone asks Bob how he liked his massage, we want him to endorse us with enthusiasm, rather than think, "I hope she acts more professional with other people." Also, our being careless with framework invites the client to do the same.

Special Considerations for Students

It's particularly common for students to bend the boundaries while they are learning their trade. Because of the dual relationships involved, bending the boundaries isn't a good idea in the long run for a serious professional practice. Still, it can be useful in the beginning to get experience, to become accustomed to working on a certain number of people a week and to practice our professional behavior as well.

Even in a practice situation, the problems of dual relationships arise, as Dianne Polseno reported in *Massage Therapy Journal*. She quotes a massage student as saying: "No one's talking about the real issues. I certainly know not to date or sleep with a client. What I don't know is how to handle the 'little things' that crop up when I massage relatives and friends. For me, this is one of the most stressful aspects of my work."*

Other students told her they had trouble establishing boundaries with friends and family. Some of the problems were:

- Difficulty in preventing a friend's massage from becoming a chatty social occasion.

- Family and friends who expect students to be "on duty" all the time.

- Holding family and friends to standard policies, such as giving adequate cancellation notice.

- Working at home and finding that a friend's session turns into a long afternoon visit.

- Feeling distressed if results aren't as good with friends or family as they are with others. (Being too subjective about our work.)

These situations could happen to any of us, but they are more common and troublesome when we are starting our practices and feeling insecure. Those "little things" that were troubling

---

*Dianne Polseno, "Ethically Speaking: Multidimensional Relationships," *Massage Therapy Journal*, Winter 1999, 113.

the massage student add up to the larger issue of claiming a professional role and setting appropriate boundaries. To avoid confusion and resentment down the road, our schools—whether massage therapy, bodywork or movement education—need to encourage students to be clear about their limits from the beginning. Most students need the support of their teachers and colleagues to set professional boundaries.

Here are some suggestions for students:

Set boundaries from the beginning: It's important for manual therapy students to set boundaries from the onset—professionalism needs to be practiced as much as technique. Before we even begin to practice sessions with friends and family, we can say, for instance, "I appreciate your acting as a guinea pig now and you'll get a free session. When I've graduated from school, I'll charge all my clients $50" (or whatever amount).

It's easier to set limits when the initial appointment is arranged—not after resentment has built because a friend has stayed for two hours after her massage. "I'll have an hour available from 2 to 3 o'clock and then I'll have to take care of some other business." It's up to us to let friends and family know the boundaries. They may not realize that they are taking advantage of us, but those "little things" can build up and add to burn-out in the future.

Treat free sessions as if they were "real" sessions—practice boundaries: It's a good way to develop professionalism and it helps the boundaries stay clear if the student treats each session as if the client were paying. Let friends and family know that they will be treated as regular clients and explain what that means: we expect to start on time, the room will be ready and we will use appropriate draping; they may talk if they want, but we won't chat back and forth as if with a friend. We can explain that this framework is helpful to us and will also help them get the most out of the session.

An added bonus is that friends and family will have the experience of seeing how professional we've become and will be more inspired to recommend us to someone else.

Becoming Friends with Clients

What happens when we try to make clients into friends? Clients feel the heart connection in our work and think that it means that they could be friends with their practitioners. Perhaps we especially like a client and think so to. Usually it's a mistake to try to change the therapeutic relationship into a social one. As mentioned before, transference makes it hard to ever have an equal relationship. On some level, clients will resist seeing their practitioners as real people with needs and flaws. There is a chance that we would always be seen as "the wise one" and that we would exploit that in some way—or that we would disappoint the client by showing our humanness. A colleague reports:

> I was thinking of accepting the invitation of a client to attend a movie together, and I knew that the client was also wanting to be friends. When I expressed my concerns to her, she said, "Oh, I know it'll be OK to be friends. I know you would never do anything that would be harmful to me." Her saying that helped me see how idealized I was in her mind. I knew we could never really be friends. I had to tell her

that it was my policy to not socialize with clients or ex-clients.

Some practitioners do socialize with clients but are always aware of their roles and responsibilities towards their clients and ex-clients. Vivien Schapera, Director of Alexander Technique of Cincinnati, says,

> We can be social but we can't show what I call our "lower selves." We can't show our pettiness, neediness, jealousies, etc. We tend to work from our higher selves, so clients tend to think we are better than we really are. We may thrive on this adulation. However, once we become friends with our clients, we may find ourselves resorting to our lower selves, in the same way as we do in the comfort of our own homes and with our closest friends.

> If we get into a difficult situation with a friend who is also a client, if they push our buttons, we have to pull ourselves out of being three years old, regardless of how "justified" we might be. We must remember that we are the practitioner, always. It never goes away. No matter how hard it is, we have to be "big," we have to be the role model, we have to be generous, we have to give the benefit of the doubt, etc.

> It's a delicate and fragile thing to have multiple roles. So if we take someone on as both a client and a friend, we are never justified in letting them down, even if they "deserve" it. That

would be like a parent letting down their child because they "deserved" it. It just doesn't work that way.

Schapera also says that she will not initiate a social invitation but will sometimes accept one from a client.

Socializing with clients should occur rarely, if at all. Feldenkrais instructor Paul Rubin says, "If you're finding a number of friends through your practice, something is out of balance. Whose needs are being met?" It's not ethical to encourage the adulation of clients or to use the offer of friendship to make them more dependent on us. Also, it can interfere with our relationship to other clients. They may hear about these friendships and become jealous or uncomfortable about the limits of our boundaries.

As with other dual relationships, people who do emotionally-oriented work cannot become friends with clients and rarely can become friends with ex-clients. Rob Bauer, Rubenfeld Synergist, says, "People get into emotional issues with Rubenfeld and transference can happen very quickly, in just one session. I don't work with friends or make friends of clients."

The Complications of Trades

It used to be, and sometimes still is, that trades were seen as a charming hippie sort of thing, a way to bypass the supposed crassness of money, a way to live more simply, bartering and trading services and goods. Trades also have the potential for being a real pain in the neck and a source of misunderstanding—especially if they are ongoing, rather than one-time. Many of the practitioners I interviewed have discontinued doing trades.

Trades are difficult because they always contain two major boundary confusions: first, there is always a dual relationship and second, there isn't the clarity and simplicity of a money exchange. We have to work harder to be sure that each side is happy with what is received and each feels the trade to be equal. We also have to work harder to establish a feeling of safety. Taking on dual roles brings confusion with it.

Like other kinds of dual relationships, trades can work if they are one-time rather than ongoing or if the work is not deep emotionally-oriented work. Some practitioners offer one trade as a way to introduce their work to the community and as a courtesy to other manual therapists.

There are ways to minimize the confusion about the exchange and also the confusion that comes from switching back and forth between roles:

Avoid trades for bodywork: Trading bodywork on an ongoing basis—a massage for a massage or other kinds of bodywork—is more likely to get unhappily complicated than other kinds of trades. Both parties are naked or partially so. Each is touching the other. It's an intimate and confusing situation that can stir up sexual issues and sexual abuse issues.

Be careful trading for any kind of service: It goes without saying that we don't trade for psychotherapy—that's not considered legitimate in the professional psychotherapy community. But what about trading for other services? One of the difficulties is in being precise. Suppose we're trading a session for two hours of house cleaning. The client's idea of how a house should look after two hours of cleaning can be different from ours. It's then very awkward to switch from a practitioner role to that of the dissatisfied customer. It's also less than desirable for a client to have such an intimate glimpse of our private lives and personal habits. A colleague says, "I don't want clients to see what's inside my car—all the junk food wrappers and clutter—much less what's inside my house."

Be clear about value when trading for goods: The happiest trades can be for various goods, particularly artwork. It's important that the value of the item be clear and agreed upon by both parties beforehand. It's more difficult if we're trading for something sight unseen, such as commissioning a piece of artwork. Even then, there can be an unexpected downside. One practitioner told me he has come to dislike a piece of art he took in trade because it reminds him of how unpleasant and difficult it was to work with the artist. Ultimately, money is simpler and cleaner.

Be clear about the exchange from the beginning: The trick with trades is to be very clear what the exchange is. Best to write it down for both parties to see. Some practitioners say they don't like doing trades because they often end up trading one of their $70 sessions for someone else's $50 session. We can trade two sessions for one or one and a half sessions for one, but the point is that we enter into the exchange knowing exactly what the trade is and that both parties are satisfied with it.

Spell out how to terminate the agreement: We need to be clear ahead of time what will happen if one of the traders decides to quit before the trade is even. Suppose a practitioner is trading Healing Touch for tap dance lessons. She's given $200 worth of Healing Touch sessions and has only received $100 worth of dance lessons. At that point, she decides she doesn't want to be the next Bojangles and doesn't need any more lessons. How do they resolve it? Since she is the one who changed her mind, does the dance teacher owe her anything? And if he does owe her the $100 balance, does he have to pay it all immediately? The details can vary, but it's best to work them out ahead of time. Putting them in writing makes sure that you both understand the terms.

Take care with boundaries: As with other dual relationships, we need to be more careful about other kinds of boundaries, rather than less careful. Our trade clients probably need an even safer environment than our regular clients. Take extra care with the framework.

Best to trade with professionals: It's easiest to trade with someone who is a professional at whatever the service or work is. Professionals will have a clear idea of their prices and how to work with clients.

Be willing to say "no": Don't trade to please or to take care of someone else and don't trade for something unneeded or unwanted. These situations are uneven from the start and can breed resentment. We also should be careful how many trades we take on at once, so that we're not working all week and ending up with no money. Remember that trades can take more energy than regular clients because of the time spent negotiating terms, as well as the likelihood of misunderstandings.

Dual Relationships with Instructors

Although this book is focused on the client/practitioner relationship, the same guidelines and ethics hold true for the instructor/student relationship. It's unethical for instructors to use the power given them by their position to benefit personally. As with the client/practitioner relationship, the focus always needs to be on the well-being of the student.

Instructors may have an even greater responsibility than practitioners to keep good boundaries. Instructors are role models
and when they overstep boundaries, it affects all their students
and not just the ones directly involved.

Some instructors may feel they are being superior or snobbish
if they don't befriend students. However, instructors who socialize with students can disrupt the whole classroom atmosphere—there can be feelings of favoritism or jealousy or other
kinds of discomfort. Good boundaries with students ultimately
serve to keep the learning environment safe. A female colleague reports:

> In my school, there was one teacher who used
> to date at least one student per class. I never
> felt comfortable taking off my clothes in front
> of him because I always felt that I was being
> evaluated as a dating prospect.

There are other ways that instructors want to be alert to boundary problems. It's probably not a good idea for an instructor to
also be a student's practitioner. As a practitioner, our attitude is
of nonjudgmental acceptance; as an instructor, our responsibility is to give constructive criticism and/or set limits on behavior. The change in roles can be confusing to both sides.

Also, if instructors actively solicit students as clients, it can be
a misuse of the power of transference. The instructor/student
dynamic is similar to the practitioner/client one—students will
usually have a hard time saying "no" to an instructor. Many
instructors are aware of this power and don't use it to influence
students to become clients. Feldenkrais assistant trainer Marcy

Lindheimer takes care to avoid the impression of recruiting students from her classes to become her private clients. When students need help with a physical issue, she always offers to refer them to other practitioners.

Taking on the role of teacher is a responsibility that extends beyond the classroom. When instructors do socialize with students—at a class party, for instance—they do not have the freedom, as Vivien Schapera says, to show their "lower selves" or to discuss personal problems. How enthusiastic can a student be if she knows that the teacher would rather be at home than teaching? How much can a student grow if he thinks the teacher prefers another student? The focus has to be on the growth of the student. Concerns about the teacher are a disruption.

Business

The ethics of selling products to clients or involving them in business deals was covered in more detail in Chapter Five on Ethics. To reiterate, there are two main problems:

- Because of transference, the client may not be as free as a non-client to refuse to buy whatever the practitioner is selling. Even a suggestion from a beloved or respected practitioner can feel like an offer the client can't refuse.

- If something goes wrong—the vitamins aren't as peppy as the client hoped, the stocks drop—the client isn't as free as a non-client to complain or treat it like a normal business arrangement.

Involving clients in other business transactions can cause resentment, even lower the client's respect for the practitioner, as well as interfering with the therapeutic relationship. It's best to avoid business transactions with clients.

Be Wary of Dual Relationships

Sometimes we're lucky and squeak by without problems despite having a dual relationship. Usually, though, they lead to anything from minor annoyances (putting extra energy into sorting out misunderstandings) to major problems (being in hot water for unethical behavior). Clients who are entangled in dual relationships with us generally don't benefit from our work as much as other clients do. There just isn't the same amount of attention and therapeutic focus.

Dual relationships can be motivated by an underlying fear about money or scarcity, and that's not a good basis for running a professional practice. Nevertheless, dual relationships will probably always be with us. It helps if we realize the problems intrinsic to their natures and take extra precautions to help the client feel safe.

The Case for Supervision & Other Forms of Self-care
✖
Chapter Ten

A career as a manual therapist requires a clear mind and a sturdy body. We have to keep our curiosity alive and our hearts open. Under necessary business expenses, we should include workshops, seminars and bodywork for ourselves. Keeping body and soul together takes a good deal of maintenance. One excellent way to stay at our best is to have ongoing supervision.

Supervision: An Idea Whose Time Has Come

"Supervision" may sound like someone telling us what to do, which may not sound appealing to manual therapists. We like to fly by the seat of our pants, we want to use our God-given intuition, we're doing just fine on our own, thank you—and we certainly don't want anyone telling us how to run our practices.

But lately, we're catching onto the fact that good supervision can nourish us and make our work easier. It can free us to do our best work. Supervision for manual therapists is an idea whose time has come.

Using supervision means using a trained professional to help us understand the dynamics of the therapeutic relationship with our clients. Supervision gives us a chance to problem-solve with an informed colleague about the best ways to help a client. It shows us those blind spots that repeatedly get in our way. However, supervision isn't psychotherapy. In supervision, we don't discuss our issues in depth, but only as they relate to our work.

Good supervisors help us see our strong points, as well as the areas in which we need to learn. Most of us would rather talk about the banks we've robbed than to talk honestly about the mistakes we've made in our work and open ourselves to possible criticism. A good supervisor knows that we all constantly make mistakes. He/she should be friendly, knowledgeable, warm and skillful. A supervisor should be in our corner, cheering on our good work and gently nudging us about our mistakes. Time with a supervisor should be like a visit with a helpful teacher, friend and/or mentor.

"But I Don't Do Psychological Work."

The most healing aspect of *any* manual therapy modality is the relationship between client and practitioner. Common sense, anecdotes and folk wisdom say it's true. Studies show it. It's the reason I'm writing this book. I can't say it enough.

Creating a therapeutic relationship is a matter of threading our way through the minefield of the client's transference and our own countertransference. It's about using clear and helpful communication with our clients and keeping clear and appropriate boundaries. And that holds true no matter what kind of manual therapy we do.

We can't avoid psychological issues, even if our intent is merely to relax muscles. Clients can get in touch with their grief, their anger, their buried and frightening memories just from physical contact (or they will defend mightily against getting in touch). We cannot avoid touching the psyche.

Even if we're not in the business of working with emotions, even if our job is just to be able to allow clients to cry and to know when to refer them to a counselor, we want to do it with grace and compassion.

"But I've Been a Bodyworker a Long Time and My Practice is Going Well."

Manual therapists who have never had supervision don't know what they're missing. Even if a practice is humming along at full tilt, it can always run more smoothly, require less energy and become more interesting. Also, even those with a prosperous practice may be making clients uncomfortable some of the time. Clients are forgiving. It's such a pleasure to be touched that they will tolerate a certain amount of clumsiness and annoying behavior if we can do a decent session. If we learn new ways to help clients feel safe and supported, we will reach new depths in our work and have more satisfying relationships with our clients.

Here are some signs that we may be complicating our work life:

- A good many "difficult" or "controlling" clients is an indication that we're not providing basic, safe framework.

- Clients who challenge our boundaries—forgetting checks, showing up late, wanting to be friends—indicate that we may be being unclear about setting limits.

- Making friends with a client more than once in a blue moon or often feeling sexually attracted to clients suggests boundary confusion.

- Frequent exhaustion at the end of the work day can be caused by blurred boundaries and unclear expectations.

Even when practices are thriving, supervision can make our work easier. When we over-identify with clients, or want to rescue them or get flummoxed dealing with difficult clients, it makes our work that much harder. Manual therapists who last over the long haul seek out plenty of support from others and find new ways to enliven their work. We've all seen people who are going full tilt one minute and heading up the burned-out or injured list the next. Supervision is a form of self-care.

A colleague reports:

> At first, I was resistant to supervision—mostly because I didn't want to expose my ignorance to someone else. After all, I'd been practicing for many years...wasn't I supposed to have most of the answers? I stumbled into a good supervisor and to make a long story short, discovered a new energy and a new interest in my clients. The annoying and demanding client became the interesting woman who was trying desperately to deal with the overwhelming experience of bodywork. The seductive man who made me a little nervous became a little boy trying to control an unfamiliar and scary situation.
>
> I became more aware of my own patterns—wanting to rescue a client in pain or being annoyed with an ungrateful client. My work became more satisfying as I understood more about what my clients needed from me in order to feel safe. And I was reassured to find that, most of the time, what I was doing was both appropriate and useful.

Supervision and Beginners: The Importance of Support

The idea of using supervision as we start our practices is relatively new. Continuing education is generally required for the technical part of our work, but until recently, the relationship aspects have been overlooked.

Schools send us out into the world with a certificate and a hearty handshake (or a soulful hug, if we live in California) and then we're on our own. Particularly in the first few years of practice, getting help can save us from making unnecessary mistakes. I wish it were a given that all manual therapists would go from school into an internship with a qualified supervisor.

Nobody tells us this in school, but it's lonely out there. We tend to work in isolation—in our homes, in a private office— and we're alone with a needy client who's in pain and looking to us for relief. Good supervision is like having a third person in the room, someone knowledgeable and compassionate, who can help us carry the load.

We often have little contact or serious discussion with other manual therapists. I've given workshops in which bodyworkers start a question with, "Maybe I'm the only one this happens to..." and then relate a common situation, such as clients being late, clients not giving enough cancellation notice or clients making sexual advances. It helps to have reassurance that others are dealing with the same dilemmas.

It also helps to have the validation of talking with a respected colleague or a group of colleagues when we are learning how to set boundaries and limits on our clients. Getting outside support and ideas is fortification for dealing with manipulative or hard-to-handle clients.

Especially in the first years of our practices, we don't know enough to know when we're in over our heads, when what a client needs is beyond our expertise or beyond the scope of our methods. Often we don't trust our intuition or know a red flag when we see one.

Here's a story that's a manual therapist's worst nightmare:

> A newly-graduated massage therapist had a client referred to him by a chiropractor. The client had swollen feet and the massage therapist was reluctant to work on them for fear of an embolism or blood clot. The client assured him that she had had that checked out and was fine. (This turned out not to be true.) In spite of the assurances, the massage therapist worked very lightly on the area. He saw the client over a period of several sessions and never quite felt comfortable working with her—even though he had her reassurances and the chiropractor's referral. Something about the client made him uneasy.

> Within days of having a massage, the client did throw an embolism and had a massive stroke and died. The massage therapist found himself, along with the chiropractor, as a defendant in a wrongful death suit. The suit against him was later dropped because it was decided that a massage therapist would not be expected to have the expertise to distinguish a dangerous medical situation. However, you can imagine the anguish the therapist experienced. And he is still feeling it. Now, every client looks like a potential lawsuit and/or someone he could potentially harm.

We don't know if supervision could have averted that disaster. It's not clear that massage caused the blood clot to dislodge, but any involvement in a death or a lawsuit is a personal disaster. A good supervisor might have noticed the practitioner's uneasiness and suggested that he make sure the client had actually been checked out by a doctor or might have urged him not to work with the client. At the least, having a supervisor would have given him someone in his corner when he was sued.

Supervision Is for Experienced Bodyworkers Too
Practitioners who have been out of school for years face the same problems as new manual therapists—the isolation, the need for validation and support and the need for help with serious issues. We need to get supervision when:

- We're working with a client who is dealing with physical or sexual abuse issues.
- We feel constantly impatient with or judgmental toward a client.
- We feel bored with our work.
- We feel ineffective or burned out.
- We can't remember why we became manual therapists.
- We're tempted by an attraction to cross our usual boundaries.
- We've been unkind to a client.

Here are some of the many ways supervision is invaluable to both the inexperienced and the seasoned practitioner:

Blind Spots: We all have less than positive things about ourselves that we put out of our awareness—ways that we might unconsciously hurt clients, ways that we might hinder their growth. We need someone who has the skill and willingness to

199

SUPERVISION CAN HELP WHEN
YOU FEEL BORED WITH YOUR WORK.

SIGH

UMM.. THAT FEELS GOOD..
A LITTLE MORE PRESSURE..

Aloha

tell us what we do not see about ourselves. Our teachers don't always do this. Nor will friends or partners/spouses. We like to think of ourselves as always caring, and it's painful to have someone, even diplomatically, point out ways we might be insensitive to others. But how else are we going to learn?

Ethics consultant Daphne Chellos says it straight out:

> Supervision is a preventive measure against abusing clients. Abuse can be unintentional as well as intentional, subtle as well as blatant. As humans, all of us can be "victims" and all of us

can be "aggressors." Our tendency is to remember violations against us and to either forget or ignore our aggressive acts. This blind spot exists as well in therapeutic relationships. A competent supervisor will notice when a therapist is being inappropriate or abusive, no matter how subtly or unintentionally and bring it to the therapist's attention.*

Keeping Confidentiality: Clients tell us their secrets. Even if they don't tell, we often guess. We know how frightened that successful, confidant-looking businessman actually is because we see the tension in his body. We sense the underlying sadness of the vivacious woman who's the life of the party. Clients confide in us about their private lives and concerns and as professionals, we are not allowed to talk about our clients with our colleagues, friends or families, and we're certainly not allowed to divulge anything they say. As Trager Approach instructor Amrita Daigle says, "If we don't have someone who we can ourselves talk with in professional confidence, we will tend to gossip about our clients." It can become a burden to carry all that pain, all those secrets. Having a supervisor, who is also bound by rules of confidentiality, gives us a way to share that burden. (Practitioners who use supervision need to have clients' permission to discuss them with their supervisors.)

Guilt: I've talked with many practitioners who feel ashamed of an instance when they used poor judgment or went outside ethical boundaries. Sometimes no harm was done to the client and sometimes the practitioner couldn't have foreseen the problem. However, these moments weigh on practitioners who strive

---

*Daphne Chellos, M.A., "Supervision in Bodywork: Borrowing a Model From Psychotherapy" in Ben Benjamin's "Bringing Boundaries to Bodywork," *Massage Therapy Journal*, Winter/1991,15

to be ethical. Talking with a trusted supervisor or mentor helps put those mistakes in perspective. A good supervisor will listen to our mistakes and errors without making us feel ashamed or incompetent.

Prejudice: How do we feel about working with other races, gay people, fat people, the chronically ill, racists, Orthodox Jews, Hindus, born-again Christians—just to name a few groups? What about people who voted for the candidate we campaigned against? Sexist men; wealthy, pampered women; angry feminists? Do any of these types of people make our hearts snap shut? We all have prejudices. Supervision will help us recognize them so that we can either get beyond our negative feelings and learn to care about the client or refer the client on to someone else.

Sorting Out Our Beliefs: We work everyday with issues of intimacy, sexuality, power, money, dependency, pain and illness. Where have we learned about these issues? What did our families teach us about touch, sickness, money or power? What does our current spiritual practice say? What does the latest self-help book say? Are all these in agreement?

None of us had a perfect childhood. No doubt we all picked up some unhealthy ideas as children about intimacy, sexuality, power, money, dependency, pain and illness. And even though we may consciously subscribe to a philosophy that is benevolent and wise, how much do our own unresolved issues affect our behavior with clients?

Supervision can help us to sort out what we truly believe. It can make us aware of the ways we continue to act on old beliefs that are no longer useful. Suppose, for instance, a bodyworker's training tells her that people can heal themselves. She'd like to believe this enlightened idea and incorporate it into her work, but she still finds herself acting as if she needs to fix her clients. Supervision could help her see how influenced she is by the cultural belief that the practitioner is responsible for healing us. Also, even though supervision isn't psychotherapy, she could learn which experiences and attitudes from her childhood are getting in her way. Supervision can help us integrate our actions with the broader and more accepting philosophies to which we usually aspire.

Help with Mentally Ill Clients

How can we distinguish a client suffering from schizophrenia from one who is not? We will find some emotionally disturbed people in our practices, and they will respond to us and our work differently than other clients. We may be baffled by their behavior, and we may do them emotional harm. Or we may not know how to take care of ourselves in working with emotionally ill clients and be harmed ourselves. A supervisor trained in psychological dynamics is a valuable resource for helping us identify and figure out what to do with mentally ill clients.

Clients with mental illness can make complaints or feel harmed, even when practitioners are ethical and careful. People with borderline personality disorder, for instance, constantly fear abandonment and feel helpless to control their lives. As caring practitioners, we may want to help a client who appears to be floundering. Yet, a person with a borderline personality disorder can exhibit extreme helplessness on the one hand and a punishing rage on the other. We may be ill-fatedly drawn to try to rescue a seemingly helpless client, only to wind up as the recipient of that person's wish to punish. For our own protection, we need help identifying mental illness.

There's a bias that says we shouldn't categorize people or label them, and therefore, we don't want to say that someone has schizophrenia or a bi-polar disorder or is clinically depressed. The rejection of labels comes from the worthy idea that we are all unique individuals and should be treated as such, and that categorizing could put people in boxes that de-humanize them.

However, we want to know whether a client is mentally ill for his or her protection as well as our own. For example, people who suffer from schizophrenia will respond differently to deep bodywork than others who are not mentally ill. People with a mental illness generally don't have the interior strength to weather a process, such as Rolfing or other kinds of transformational work, that can strip away defenses. Ordinary folk seek out that kind of work in order to experience a deeper part of themselves. For disturbed people, who feel blank or chaotic behind their social exterior, such work can be uncomfortable and disorienting. An experienced supervisor can help us identify signs of mental illness and judge whether our work will be beneficial to the prospective client:

> Years ago when I was doing a form of emotionally-oriented bodywork without much training, I had a client who baffled me. She was a high-powered, successful businesswoman who looked and dressed the part; however, during a session, she never seemed to access anything but superficial emotions.

At my suggestion, she attended a personal growth workshop in which I was assisting. At one point, she was working with the main teacher, as the rest of us watched. As she became more emotional, she also became more irrational and almost incoherent: she began to unravel like an old sweater. I was surprised to see that what was underneath her polished exterior was a very disturbed confusion. The teacher worked to help her find her way back to an accustomed state of mind that was comfortable to her. After that workshop, I never saw the client again.

Support for Our Intuition

Many manual therapists use their intuition to understand how best to work with a client. Intuition is a useful gift, but sometimes it fails us; sometimes clients slip beneath the radar of our intuition. We misread them and fail to offer them the kind of support they need. That failure can confuse and demoralize a practitioner, who may then begin to mistrust his intuition. A good supervisor can help us see the reasons we didn't understand the client and educate us about how best to use our intuitive side.

And the #1 Reason for Getting Supervision: I know it's a little late to say this but—good boundaries can't be learned from reading a book. We have to experience them. We have to know how they feel, how safe we feel when we are working with someone who is clear and careful with boundaries. It's a matter of getting the solid feeling of good boundaries inside us.

A book can give us an idea of why it's important to be professional, but we can't learn it all from a book. Many of us have
had a few teachers along the way who were careless or uneducated about boundaries, and we need a remedial experience.
In the same way that we can't be a really good massage therapist if we've never experienced massage, we can't have excellent
boundaries with our clients unless we've had the experience of
being on the other side, of being a client with a good supervisor. Sorry...but there's no way around it. If we aspire to a high
level of professionalism, we need the good modeling that a
compassionate professional trained in transference and countertransference can provide.

Choosing a Supervisor

What should we look for in a supervisor? In order to learn
decent boundaries, we're best off choosing someone with whom
we don't have any other kind of relationship, someone with
whom we're not already bending the boundaries. That makes
sense, doesn't it? A friend may be a skilled psychologist but she
wouldn't be an objective supervisor because there's a dual relationship. (See Chapter Nine on Dual Relationships.)

We want to find someone who is aware of transference and
countertransference, fundamental therapeutic dynamics and
abuse issues. The psychotherapist or counselor we choose also
needs to be respectful of the manual therapies and, ideally, has
been a client or has some other reason to be a fan of our work.
We may also be lucky enough to find a manual therapist who
has a strong background in psychology.

A manual therapist's supervisor has to understand the powerful dynamics that come into play when we touch people. Since

hands-on work can readily bring up both deep longings and prior abuse issues, a supervisor should understand that the need for manual therapy clients to feel safe may be even greater than "talk therapy" clients' need for safety.

A supervisor should be someone with whom we have a formal business relationship—a contract to meet at a certain time and pay X for the consultation. Occasionally asking a friend or colleague a question isn't the same as having an ongoing relationship with a professional who is responsible for helping us learn. It takes time for someone to get a clear picture of our strong and weak areas. A casual supervisory relationship with a friend or colleague doesn't give him enough permission to confront us about our blind spots.

What Kind of Supervision is Best?

The question isn't whether or not we should have supervision, but what kind and how often. Practitioners who are serious about their work will probably need to seek different kinds of supervision at one time or another. Many experienced practitioners still make use of supervision, mentoring and peer group formats for their learning. As we gain experience, we may not need help as frequently as we did when we were starting out, but none of us outgrow the need for outside help and feedback.

With E-mail and inexpensive long-distance rates, neither our mentor nor our supervisor needs to be in our city. They just need to be someone we respect, who has enthusiasm for and knowledge of our kind of manual therapy and who is interested in working with us. Supervision can take various forms and there are pros and cons for each.

Group Supervision: Less expensive than individual supervision, it's great for dealing with isolation. Group supervision is an excellent way to learn the norms of our work and gather ideas about the ways others work with issues that are common to all of us. It is also good support and helps us see that we're not alone or unusual in the problems we're having.

People who stay with this work over the long haul usually have a group or community that strongly supports and educates them—it's vital to the health of our practices. Some practitioners create their own group by finding a good supervisor and bringing together interested colleagues.

Individual Supervision: This type of supervision may cost more per session but can be tailored to an individual's specific issues. Private work is also better for people who wouldn't feel comfortable revealing their insecurities and mistakes to a group.

Peer Groups: It is possible to meet as a group of practitioners to discuss common issues without a supervisor. Peer groups are not supervised by any of the members and have different benefits from supervision. Nan Narboe, clinical social worker and boundaries expert, says:

> There are things that only your peers will tell you and that you can only hear from your peers. For instance, if our supervisor praises a piece of work we do, we may assume she's "just being nice." If we hear the same praise from our peers, we tend to believe it. There are times, however, when individual supervision is best. There are things that only your supervisor will tell you and that you can only hear from your supervisor—such as where your blind spots are.

Peer groups are an excellent and inexpensive way to get support and learn from others, but they can't substitute for individual supervision.

Mentoring: This form of support is an agreement with a more experienced colleague that she or he will be available to answer our questions. It can be an informal arrangement and is often unpaid. It may be as simple as, "Let me take you to lunch and get the benefit of your years as a bodyworker." Everyone graduating from manual therapy training needs a mentor. It should be a given that we're not expected to start a practice without help and support.

Mentoring usually addresses less complex issues than supervision. It's very good for business and practice-building kinds of questions—such as the value of an answering service or the pros and cons of working out of our homes.

Other Kinds of Self-Care

Quality Bodywork

Getting good bodywork for ourselves is vital. Just having our buddy work on us every now and then isn't enough. We need to go to practitioners with whom we don't have another relationship and who are more experienced and skilled than we are. If we work with the most skilled and experienced manual therapists around, we will benefit in many ways: we will learn from them, our bodies will appreciate the good work and we will be inspired—our faith in bodywork will be renewed.

Clients can tell when we've gotten stale and burned out, when we're plodding along in a rote way. The antidote is once again discovering the delight and miracle of our work and the way a good session can change our outlook on life.

Workshops and Seminars

Workshops and seminars can be revitalizing. There is the danger of thinking of ourselves as "instant experts" after attending one workshop. (See Chapter Two on Boundaries.) However, there is nothing that can energize us like the excitement of being in a room full of other dedicated practitioners or learning a new slant on our work. Attending workshops is a necessary part of keeping interest in our work alive.

Taking Care of Ourselves

To forestall burn-out, manual therapists need to take good care of themselves and that means getting help from others. Good supervision helps us be more elegantly and crisply professional. Sharing with someone else what really goes on in our offices, what pushes our buttons, where our hearts get shut down—someone who can help us find our way through this complex and demanding work—is crucial to the health of our practices.

Being a client ourselves can renew our enthusiasm for our work and give us more vitality. Supervision, peer support and workshops take away the isolation and depletion that kill our interest in our work. Our professional lives are more rewarding when we find ways to keep our interest alive and to be kinder to ourselves.

Discussion Questions for the Classroom

With questions that require discussion, students may be divided into small groups to facilitate everyone's participation and then brought back into the larger group with each small group reporting their discussion. Teachers need to caution students not to reveal the identity of any clients or professionals in the stories they tell.

Chapter One — The Educated Heart

1. Have students describe, in as much detail as they can, their ideal session both as a client and as a practitioner. What are the important elements? After discussion, what did they add to their description from other people's comments?

2. What is the student's understanding of the idea that memories and old feelings get locked in the body and can be released through touch by a massage therapist or bodyworker or through movement facilitation by a movement teacher? Ask them to describe their own experiences.

3. Have students describe a time when a manual therapist or other kind of professional (doctor, chiropractor, etc.) was authentic with them in a way that was therapeutic and a time when a professional was "authentic" (perhaps too casual or too self-revealing, for instance) in a way that was not therapeutic.

Chapter Two — Boundaries: Protective Circles

1. For the student: You work in a health spa as a massage

therapist. Clients frequently invite you to join them in a social activity, such as having lunch or attending a party. Some clients you would like to get to know better. Others, you wouldn't. What are the boundary and ethical considerations in deciding what to do?

2. A client says she is involved in an unhappy affair with a married man who will never leave his wife. The relationship is going nowhere. She says she doesn't know what to do and she seems confused and very upset. How does the student respond? (Role playing would be useful here: the student may know what to say from a thoughtful distance but not in the immediacy of the moment.)

3. Have students role-play keeping the focus on the client in this situation: You are pregnant and just starting to show. Your client begins to ask you questions —your due date, your marital status, your health status, etc. How do you respond? How much do you tell the client? What concerns might the client have? (Don't forget that a male student can play a pregnant woman also.)

Chapter Three — Client/Practitioner Dynamics: The Power Imbalance

1. Ask students to think of a situation with a manual therapist in which they were the client and they didn't tell the practitioner to stop or question what he was doing, as they might have ordinarily. (If they haven't had enough experience with other manual therapists, make it any kind of professional.) Share with the class. If they had been that practitioner, what could they have said or done to make it easier for them, as the client, to assert themselves?

2. Role-play working with a difficult, picky client. Make sure the "client" gives feedback about how the student's response felt and what helped or would have helped him/her feel less anxious.

3. Clients get crushes on practitioners. What are the signs that a client has a crush, and how does the student feel about clients having a crush? How will she/he handle it?

Chapter Four — Framework: Nuts and Bolts

1. Have students discuss which components of framework are particularly important to them when they are clients. Has it ever spoiled a session for them when a professional was careless about one of these components?

2. As a prospective client of a manual therapist or of any kind of professional, when have students been positively or negatively influenced by the initial phone conversation? What made the difference? When have they been positively or negatively influenced by the appearance of an office or the practitioner's initial presentation of him or herself?

3. Ask students to role-play what they would say to (1) a prospective client who wants to know the benefits of their work, (2) a client who wants to give them a lengthy history over the phone, (3) a client who says she can't afford their prices but that she'd really like a session, and (4) a client who wants a guarantee about the results of their work. Have the person who plays the client give feedback about how effective the responses of the "practitioner" were.

Chapter Five — Ethics: From Theory to Practice

1. You meet someone at a party to whom you are attracted and that person wants to make an appointment with you. Is it alright to do that? Have students indicate where they stand on this issue by designating one end of the room as #1, they feel strongly that it's alright, and the other end as #10, they feel strongly that it's not alright. Then ask students to stand at one end or the other or

somewhere in between to show their position on the question. Ask students at various positions to explain their reasons.

2. What prejudices does the student have; what kind of person would be hard for him or her to work with? What will the student do when such a person is a prospective client? (It may be hard to get in touch with prejudices.) Are there any groups of people that the student thinks all act alike or groups with whom the student wouldn't want to socialize?

3. How do the students feel about selling products to clients? What are their considerations?

Chapter Six — Sexual Issues: Protecting Our Clients

1. Remembering confidentiality, have students describe an incident when they were clients and felt that the practitioner may not have had sexual intentions, but was insensitive in his/her behavior.

2. The argument that some practitioners use to justify dating clients is, "After all, we're both adults." What do your students think about that argument? How does the issue of transference affect the ethics of dating clients?

3. How do students feel about dating an ex-client? What are the considerations involved?

Chapter Seven — Sexual Issues: Protecting Ourselves

1. For both male and female students: role-play a situation in which a client on the table wants sexual services.

2. Use a "fishbowl" format in which one group sits in a circle and talks while a second group sits in a circle around them and only listens. In a fishbowl, time is allotted for the inner circle's discus-

sion and then time is allotted for the outer circle to talk about their feelings and experiences while they were listening to the inner circle discussion. The outer circle is cautioned not to positively or negatively comment on any comments made in the inner circle or engage in arguments.

Have men and women take turns being the inner and outer circles and have each discuss their fears related to sexual issues, first as clients, then as practitioners.

3. How do massage therapy students feel about the public's confusion of legitimate massage therapy with prostitutes? What do they do when friends or acquaintances make jokes or insinuations?

Chapter Eight — Getting Comfortable with Money

1. Have students complete the sentence, "Money is _____." Write the responses on the board. Have students identify which responses resonate with them. What can students do to change any unhealthy responses with which they may identify?

2. Have students write an imaginary ad for themselves as a practitioner—what personal qualities and professional skills would they highlight?

3. Role-play the situation of having a new client ask the practitioner at the end of a session if he can mail his check later.

Chapter Nine — Dual Relationships: Wearing Many Hats

1. Have students describe any difficulty they have had working with someone on a trade basis. What would they do differently next time? If they've done trades without having a problem (having a misunderstanding or receiving work that isn't top quality,

for example), what did they do that helped the trade be problem-free?

2. Have the students already experienced problems working with friends or family? What can they do to lessen those problems?

3. Have students role-play how they will set limits with friends and family before they begin working with them.

Chapter Ten —The Case for Supervision and Other Forms of Self-Care

1. While they are in school, students often don't realize how isolated and depleted they can get as practitioners. They don't always realize how many confusing interpersonal relationship questions will come up in working with clients. Have them make concrete plans to take care of themselves after they graduate.

2. The idea of supervision is still a new one for manual therapists. How do students feel about it? What are their pros and cons?

3. Practitioners often say that they don't have "enough" money to afford self-care—to attend a stimulating workshop, pay for quality bodywork or get supervision. Have students discuss their answers to "Money is_____." (See Chapter Eight questions) in relation to their feelings about whether or not they can afford self-care.

Acknowledgments*

There's no exaggeration in saying that this book couldn't have been written without Nan Narboe. Many years ago, she planted the seed for it and in recent years, she performed herculean tasks to make it possible—non-stop support, brilliant editing and wise counsel. *The Educated Heart* is very much her book also.

A good editor has to know when to treat your work as if it were a fragile baby bird and when to offer scalpel-sharp clarity. Nan is not only a great editor, she is a skilled clinician *and* she is a passionate advocate of clean professional boundaries. I was blessed to find such a helper.

Others came along to help as the book progressed. Clarissa Pinkola Estés stepped in at just the right moment with her kind-hearted support and good words. She is truly *la madrina*, the godmother, of this book.

I had excellent artistic help with this book. The cartoonist, Mari Gayatri Stein, is as delightful as her amazing and quirky cartoons. I think of her dogs, cats and mice and their whimsical antics whenever I want to smile. I'm so pleased to know Mari and have her wonderful work in this book.

Jennifer Woodhull, wordsmith supreme and faithful friend, added her considerable skills to the marketing and back cover copy. The artist, Dolph Smith, was most generous in allowing me to use his beautiful work for the book cover. I'm also grateful to the graphic artists, Amy Sharp, who created a beautiful cover and Kelli Glazier, who skillfully designed the good-looking text of the book and the back cover.

*Special thanks to all the manual therapists who were interviewees and/or chapter readers. They are listed in the Special Acknowledgments, page 221.

Anne Hoff provided quality proofreading that laid the groundwork and Jennifer Werner helped out wonderfully in the frantic last days.

Ben Bledsoe, who has been the man of the hour for me before, graciously stepped in once again. His crucial fine-tuning and support at the 11th hour were greatly reassuring.

I am appreciative of Les Kertay, Ph.D., clinical psychologist and Advanced Certified Rolfer, for the concept, used throughout this book, of specialness as a red flag. He contributed the idea of secrecy as a sign of problems also.

Sharon Burch, author of *Recognizing Health and Illness: Pathology for Massage Therapists and Bodyworkers,* was generous with her time and invaluable advice.

Colleagues—Teachers and Friends

I've been blessed with extraordinary bodywork teachers—compassionate, wise and skilled. In the world of Rolfing, they were Peter Melchior, Tom Wing, Nicholas French and the late great Stacey Mills. I knew Peter and Stacey when they were instructors with the Rolf Institute. Peter is now an instructor with the Guild for Structural Integration and Stacey Mills was a teacher for the Guild before her retirement.

In more recent years, I have been touched by the staff of the Rosen Method Center Southwest in Santa Fe who came into my life like angels. They deserve special tribute: I am grateful to the wise and generous Sandra Wooten for her fierce dedication to her work and for her open-hearted teachings. Cameron Hough, full of light and grace, has honored me with her steadfast willingness to help me along my path. My friend, the elegant and vastly-talented Julia Martin, has simply been a blessing in my life. And I have a special place in my heart for the compassionate, knowing and always delightful, Karen Anderson. Her strong and life-affirming spirit brought me back from the edge many times. My life is so much richer because of the presence of each of these fine women.

My fellow students and colleagues from the Southwest Rosen Intensives have sustained me. Some gave special help for this book: my friend Jennifer Cook saved the day; Alan Fogel's help was greatly appreciated; and over the months, Patty Owens and Marjorie Huebner gave much-needed support. Felipe Ortega's words made a difference. The crew from Ghost Ranch (and thereabouts) lifted me and carried me along.

Every bodyworker who has supported me or been my friend has contributed to this book and while I can't thank all of them, here are a few notables: Jill Breslau, Helen Luce and Robert Litman, Barbara Featherstone, Marekah Stewart, Leslee McKnight-McCallum, Wayne Knerr, Sandra Waggener, Theresa Lumiere, Lee Phillips, Sherri Cassuto, Sharon DeCelle, Bobbie Donnelly, Jim Rule, Gene Elliott and Nancy Dennis.

Bonnie Gintis, D.O., contributed useful information. Carol Risher, psychotherapist, helped with the early development of some of this material. Adele Balton, CPA, is an angel.

I give special thanks to Karen Craig, director of the Massage Institute of Memphis, for being constantly available with resources and excellent advice. Diane Bauer is the good massage therapist mentioned in the Robbie story in the Frameworks Chapter.

Friends and Family and Helpers

It tickles me that old friends—some of them since kindergarten—had a hand in helping with this book. They are Robbie McQuiston, Suzanne Henley, Blanche Deaderick and Barbara Holden. I'm very grateful to the sinfully talented Suzanne Henley for suggesting the basic concept for the cover and being the photographer for the back cover picture.

Soon after beginning to write this book, I saw how crucial it is to have support for such a project. A few of the people attentive to me were Dr. James and Suzanne Millican, Ben Bledsoe and Susan Herron, Anne and Sid Lasky, Charlotte Schultz, Peggy Munson, Maura Marini, Ellen Klyce, Ciretha Barton, Rodney Rastall, Tom and Ginger Jeanes, Robert Ervin and Gene Aldridge. I'm grateful to the people at Prescott who kept asking, "How's that book coming?" Tom Walsh gave aid and comfort above and beyond the call of duty; Tom is the embodiment of brotherly love.

The extraordinary counselor Janet Zimmerman helped over the years by providing enough light that I could see where I was going and enough warmth that I cared whether I got there.

Cousin Ellen Rolfes had excellent counsel and wisdom to pass on and was a major cheering section. I had great support and practical advice from my brother and sister-in-law, John and Margaret. Had they known what I was up to, I know my other brother and sister-in-law, Bill and Ellen, would have thought it was a good idea. Uncle Malcolm made it all possible and for that, I will be forever grateful.

SPECIAL ACKNOWLEDGMENTS

I am grateful to the people listed below who were interviewees and/or chapter readers for this book. All gave valuable assistance and inspired me with their thoughtfulness and dedication. None of these good people are responsible for or necessarily in agreement with the opinions expressed in this book.

Rob Bauer, CSW: Master Rubenfeld Synergist; Senior Faculty Member and Supervisor, Rubenfeld Center; Salem, New York

Ben Benjamin, Ph.D: Ethics author; President of Muscular Therapy Institute; Cambridge, Massachusetts

Kathryn Benson: Clinical Consultant; Ethics teacher; Nashville, Tennessee

Mary Bernau-Eigen: Certified Advanced Rolfer; Cranial-sacral therapist; Milwaukee, Wisconsin

Heida Brenneke, M.A., LMP: Owner and director of Brenneke School of Massage; Seattle, Washington

Sue Brenner: Director, Rosen Center East; Westport, Connecticut

Rose Bronec: Co-director of training, Urbana Center for Alexander Technique; Urbana, Illinois

Gary Brownlee: Certified Trager Approach Instructor; Manhattan Beach, California

Carol Burke, M.S., CRNP: Former Director of Education, Baltimore School of Massage; Baltimore, Maryland

Marie Carbone: Mill Valley, California

Olivia Cheever: Certified Feldenkrais practitioner; licensed MT; licensed psychotherapist; Newton, Massachusetts

Daphne Chellos: Psychotherapist; Ethics consultant; Boulder, Colorado

Melissa Chipman, LMT: Ithaca, New York

Amrita Daigle: Certified Trager Approach instructor; Quebec City, Quebec

Kirsten DeMier, MT: Northern California

Barbara Tift Featherstone: Lomi School associate; Body-centered psychotherapist; Redding, Washington

Alan Fogel, Ph.D.: Professor of Psychology, University of Utah; Rosen Method bodywork student; Salt Lake City, Utah

Linda Frisone: Rosen Method bodywork practitioner; Santa Fe, New Mexico

Sandy Fritz: Owner, Health Enrichment Center; LaPeer, Michigan

Cindy Getchonis, LMT: Trager Approach practitioner; Instructor, Finger Lakes School of Massage; Ithaca, New York

William J. Greenberg, LMT: AMTA National Grievance Chair; Fairfield, Connecticut

Karna Handy: Membership Services Director, Rolf Institute; Boulder, Colorado

Annie Hartzog: Certified Rolfer; Tulsa, Oklahoma

Natasha Heifitz: Certified Trager Approach instructor; Fairfax, California

Joseph Heller: Founder of Hellerwork; Mt. Shasta, California

Anna Johnson-Chase: Certified Teacher of Feldenkrais Method, Assistant Trainer; former Chair, Ethics Committee, Feldenkrais Guild of N.A.; Milwaukee, Wisconsin

Arnold Katz, LMT: Boston, Massachusetts

Les Kertay, Ph.D.: Clinical psychologist; Chair, Ethics Committee, Rolf Institute; Certified Advanced Rolfer; Chattanooga, Tennessee

Robert K. King: Founder and president, Chicago School of Massage Therapy; Past president, AMTA; Chicago, Illinois

Carole LaRochelle: Certified Rolfer; Kent, Washington

David Lauterstein: Co-Director, The Lauterstein-Conway Massage School; Austin, Texas

Lucy Liben, M.S., LMT: Dean for Academic Affairs, Swedish Institute; New York, New York

Marcy Lindheimer: Feldenkrais Practitioner; Assistant Trainer; Former Chair, Feldenkrais Guild Ethics Committee; New York, New York

Til Luchau: Advanced Certified Rolfer; Co-ordinator, Foundations of Bodywork, Rolf Institute; Boulder, Colorado

Michael Maskornick: Certified Advanced Rolfer; Bellingham, Washington

Edward W. Maupin, Ph.D.: Psychologist; President, International Professional School of Bodywork; San Diego, California

Leslee McKnight-McCallum, LMT: EMT-Paramedic, Instructor/Coordinator; Memphis, Tennessee

Margaret Avery Moon: Director, Desert Institute of the Healing Arts; Tucson, Arizona

Thomas Myers: Advanced Certified Rolfer; Anatomy Instructor, Rolf Institute; Scarborough, Maine

Laurie Owen, LMP: Olympia, Washington

Jim Pearson, LMT: Coronado, California

Lee Phillips, MT: Levittown, Pennsylvania

Dianne Polseno, LPN, LMT: Ethics Columnist for *Massage Therapy Journal*; North Smithfield, Rhode Island

Marion Rosen: Founder, Rosen Institute; Berkeley, California

Paul Rubin: Feldenkrais teacher and Certified Trainer; San Francisco, California

Vivien Schapera: Director of Alexander Technique of Cincinnati; Cincinnati, Ohio

Bill Scholl: Trager Approach instructor; Austin, Texas

Jan Schwartz: Education Director, Desert Institute of the Healing Arts; Tucson, Arizona

Ethel Scrivener: Rhythmic Massage Therapist; Certified Teacher of the Alexander Technique; Memphis, Tennessee

Kristina Shaw: Director, Healing Hands School of Massage; Philadelphia, Pennsylvania

Chris Smith: Director of Education, Colorado School of Healing Arts; Lakewood, Colorado

Cherie Sohnen-Moe: Author; Ethics trainer; Business consultant; Tucson, Arizona

Gail Stewart: Director, reSource bodywork training program; Berkeley, California

Theresa E. Stogner, P.T: Certified Feldenkrais Teacher; Atlanta, Georgia

Kylea Taylor, M.S., MFCC: Author, *Ethics of Caring;* Santa Cruz, California

Diana L. Thompson, LMP: Author, *Hands Heal: Documentation for Massage Therapy;* Seattle, Washington

Nancy Forst Williamson: Certified Feldenkrais practitioner; Alexander teacher; former chair Feldenkrais Guild Ethics committee; Lincoln, Nebraska

Charles Wiltsie, LMT: Ethics Instructor for men; Higganum, Connecticut

Chloe Wing: Alexander teacher; director, The Musician's Body; New York, New York

Sandra Wooten: Director, Rosen Method Center Southwest; Orinda, California

Dwight Zieman: Director, Cayce-Reilly School; Virginia Beach, Virginia

Special thanks to: **Heather Merritt, Rebecca Naifeh, Sabrina Johnson,** and **Angela Watkins,** who helped while they were students at the Massage Institute of Memphis.

Resources

The following list of schools and associations is by no means a comprehensive list of manual therapy schools and associations. They are resources for the reader who would like to contact organizations whose methods are mentioned in this book.

Alexander Technique
Alexander Technique International
Cambridge, Massachusetts
(617)497-2242
www.ATI-net.com

North American Society of Teachers of the Alexander Technique
Minneapolis, Minnesota
(800)473-0620
www.alexandertech.com

Aston-Patterning
Aston-Patterning
Incline Village, Nevada
(775)831-8228

Craniosacral Therapy
American CranioSacral Therapy Association
Palm Beach Gardens, Florida
(800)311-9204

Feldenkrais
The Feldenkrais Guild
Albany, Oregon
(800)775-2118
www.feldenkrais.com

Healing Touch
Healing Touch International
Lakewood, Colorado
(303)989-7982
www.healingtouch.net

Hellerwork
Hellerwork International
Mt. Shasta, California
(530)926-2500
www.hellerwork.com

Polarity Therapy
American Polarity Therapy Association
Boulder, Colorado
(303)545-2080
www.PolarityTherapy.org

Reiki
American Reiki Masters Assn.
Lake City, Florida
(904)755-9638

The Reiki Alliance
Cataldo, Idaho
(208)783-3535

Rosen Method
Rosen Method,
Berkeley Center
(510)845-6606
www.mcn.org/B/rosen

Rosen Center East
Westport, Connecticut
(203)226-0464
www.rosencentereast.com

Rosen Method Center
  Southwest
Santa Fe, New Mexico
(505)982-7149
www.mcn.org/b/rosen/wrc.html

Rubenfeld Synergy
  Method
Rubenfeld Synergy Center
New York, New York
(800)747-6897
http://members.aol.com
rubenfeld/synergy/index.html

St. John's
  Neuromuscular
  Therapy Method
St. John's Seminars
Largo, Florida
(888)NMT-HEAL

Structural Integration
Guild for Structural Integration
Boulder, Colorado
(303)447-0122
www.rolfguild.org

Rolf Institute of Structural
  Integration
Boulder, Colorado
(800)530-8875
www.rolf.org

Trager Work
Trager Institute
Mill Valley, California
(415)388-2688
www.trager.com

Zero Balancing
Zero Balancing
Capitola, California
(831)476-0665
www.zerobalancing.com

Other
Hakomi Integrative Somatics
Boulder, Colorado
(303)447-3290

GLOSSARY

✖

Author's Note about Boundaries, Framework and Ethics: There's a good deal of overlap between boundaries, framework and ethics. Some issues, such as confidentiality, fall within all three. Some, such as whether or not we have answering machines, clearly only belong in one category—in this case, framework. I hope that no student is ever tested closely on these differentiations or on which issue goes where. There is simply too much overlap and in a way, it does not matter how we classify a behavior, as long as we make good judgments about it.

Boundary: As used in this context, a boundary relates to keeping within the professional role and the contract. For instance, not socializing with clients or not taking on a problem that is beyond the practitioner's training. Boundaries define what will and will not occur between practitioner and client in accordance with maintaining a therapeutic relationship.

One definition of boundary is the energetic and emotional space around the practitioner and the client. In this case, boundary confusion would mean the practitioner's inability to distinguish between his/her feelings and the client's. Although this is a legitimate way to talk about boundaries, it's not the way the term is used in this book. Here, "boundaries" means all the ways that relationships with clients are defined as professional.

Clinician: A licensed psychotherapist—generally a psychiatrist, psychologist or clinical social worker—who is knowledgeable about interpersonal dynamics.

Contract: The contract with the client, although it can be a written contract, is more commonly implicit—an implied agreement describing what the practitioner will and will not do, as defined by her/his training and by the ethical standards of her/his profession. A contract also implies that the manual therapist's services are exchanged for fees, goods or services from the client.

Countertransference: When the practitioner unconsciously reacts to the client by projecting (transferring) unresolved feelings, needs and issues—usually from childhood—onto the client.

Dual Relationship: An alliance other than the contractual therapeutic one with the client—such as social, familial, business or any other relationship that is outside the contractual role of the practitioner.

Emotionally-oriented bodywork: Manual therapy that is based on the concept that physical tension and restriction are related to a client's patterns of unconscious holding that the client has adopted, often early in life, to cope with his/her surroundings. The practitioner seeks to help the client release these unconscious holdings. Also called transformational work.

Framework: All the prerequisites and the conditions that allow effective manual therapy to occur. It includes not only the explicit ground rules of consistency in fees, hours and location but also the implicit ground rules of confidentiality and keeping the focus on the client.

Manual therapies: Any professional method that involves the practitioner touching the physical or the energetic body of the client for the purpose of facilitating awareness, health and wellbeing. Includes massage therapists, bodyworkers, movement educators, practitioners of the Oriental methods, emotionally-oriented bodyworkers, and practitioners who work with energy fields.

Manual therapist: A professional practitioner of any kind of work who touches the client's body (or touches the energetic body of the client) for the purpose of facilitating awareness, health and well-being.

Mentor: A trusted colleague who takes on the role of providing guidance and education for a new or less experienced practitioner. A mentor is generally helpful in advising on both the details of establishing oneself as a professional and also the broader aspects of taking on a professional role or a role as a particular kind of practitioner.

Peer group: A group of colleagues who meet on a consistent basis to discuss common issues related to their professional lives, to share information and strategies as well as to receive emotional support. A peer group is not lead by any one member.

Supervision: An arrangement with a professional trained in interpersonal dynamics to advise a practitioner about the relationship aspects of his work. Supervision includes clarifying clients' transference issues and the practitioner's countertransference issues, suggesting effective interventions, as well as identifying the practitioner's vulnerabilities and areas of strength.

Therapeutic relationship: Any relationship can be therapeutic but in this context what is meant is a relationship between practitioner and client that is focused on the well-being of the client and is contractual.

Transference: When the client unconsciously reacts to the practitioner by projecting (transferring) unresolved feelings, needs and issues—usually from childhood—onto the practitioner.

Transformational work: Any manual therapy can be transformational. However, in the context of this book, transformational work means manual therapy that is based on the concept that tension and restriction in the physical body are related to patterns of unconscious holding that the client has adopted, often early in life, to cope with her/his surroundings. It is based on the concept that helping the client access and release unconscious holdings can bring about a lasting positive change in the client's emotional and physical state.

Related Reading

Benjamin, Ben, Ph.D. *Massage and Bodywork with Survivors of Abuse*, Cambridge, Massachusetts, 1995. Contact: 617/576-0777.

Bertherat, Therese and Carol Bernstein. *The Body Has Its Reasons*, New York: Pantheon Books, 1977.

Borysenko, Joan. *Minding the Body, Mending the Mind*, Bantam Press, 1988.

Burch, Sharon, MSN. *Recognizing Health and Illness: Pathology for Massage Therapists and Bodyworkers*, Lawrence, Kansas: Health Positive!, 785/843-5884. E-mail: 4health@idir.net.

Cohen, Bonnie Bainbridge. *Sensing, Feeling, Action: The Experiential Anatomy of Body-Mind Centering*, 1993, The School for Body-Mind Centering. Contact: 413/256-8615.

Cousins, Norman. *The Healing Heart*, New York: W. W. Norton & Co., 1983.

Dossey, Larry, M.D. *Healing Words: The Power of Prayer and the Practice of Medicine*, New York: HarperSan Francisco, 1993.

Duff, Kat. *The Achemy of Illness*, New York: Pantheon Books, 1993.

Dychwald, Ken. *Body-Mind*, New York: Jove Publications, Inc., 1977.

Evans, Maja, CMT. *The Ultimate Handbook: Self-Care for Bodyworkers and Massage Therapists*, Laughing Duck Press, 1992. Contact: 301/540-5877.

Feldenkrais, Moshe. *Awareness Through Movement*, New York: Harper and Row, 1972.

Ford, Clyde, DC. *Compassionate Touch*, Simon and Schuster, 1993.

Frank, Jerome D., Ph.D., M.D., and Julia B. Frank, M.D. *Persuasion and Healing*, Johns Hopkins University Press, 1993.

Grafelman, Tricia. *Graf's Anatomy*, Cottrell Printing, 1999. Contact: 703-629-8339.

Grafelman, Tricia. *Graf's Physiology*, Cottrell Printing, 1999. Contact: 703/629-8339.

Herman, Judith L., M.D. *Trauma and Recovery*, New York: Harper Collins Publishers, Inc., 1992.

Juhan, Deane. *Job's Body: A Handbook for Bodywork*, New York: Station Hill Press, Inc., 1987.

Keleman, Stanley. *Emotional Anatomy*, Berkeley, California: Center Press, 1985.

King, Robert. *Performance Massage*, Champaign, Illinois: Human Kinetics, 1993. Contact: 800/747-4457.

Krieger, Delores. *Living The Therapeutic Touch*, New York: Dodd, Mead & Co., 1987.

Kurtz, Ron. *Body-Centered Psychotherapy, The Hakomi Method*, LifeRhythm (Press), 1990. Contact: P.O. Box 806, Mendocino, California 95460.

Lauterstein, David. *Putting the Soul Back in the Body: A Manual of Imaginative Anatomy for Massage Therapists*, Lauterstein-Conway Massage School, Austin, Texas, 1985. Contact: 800/474-0852.

Lowen, Alexander. *The Betrayal of the Body*, Macmillan Publishing Co., 1967.

Narboe, Nan, L.C.S.W. *Working with What You Can't Get Your Hands On*, Portland, Oregon.: Nan Narboe, 1985. Contact: 503/221-9760

Pert, Candace B., Ph.D. *Molecules of Emotion*, New York: Touchstone, Simon and Schuster, 1997.

Remen, Rachel Naomi. *Kitchen Table Wisdom*, New York: Riverhead Books, 1996.

Rosen, Marion and Sue Brenner. *The Rosen Method of Movement*, Berkeley, CA: North Atlantic Books, 1991.

Shealy, C. Norman, M.D., Ph.D. ed. *The Complete Family Guide to Alternative Medicine*, Barnes and Noble, 1996.

Smith, Fritz Frederick M.D. *Inner Bridges*, Atlanta: Humanics New Age, 1986.

Sohnen-Moe, Cherie M. *Business Mastery*, Tucson: Sohnen-Moe Associates, 1997. Contact: 800/ 786-4774

Taylor, Kylea. *The Ethics of Caring*, Santa Cruz, CA: Hanford Mead, 1995. Contact: 831/459-6855.

Thompson, Diana, LMP. *Hands Heal: Documentation for Massage Therapy*, Seattle: Diana Thompson, 1993. Contact: 800/989-4743, ext. 7.

Trager, Milton. *Trager Mentastics: Movement as a Way to Agelessness*, New York: Station Hill Press, Inc., 1987.

Wooten, Sandra. *Touching the Body, Reaching the Soul*, Santa Fe: 1995. Contact: 505/988-2602. E-mail: sw.touch@ix.netcom.com.

INDEX

�֎

NOTES

THE EDUCATED HEART

To order *The Educated Heart* call
☎ 877/327-0600 (toll free).
Monday-Thursday, 9 a.m. to 5 p.m. (CST).
Major Credit Cards accepted.
Ask about volume discounts.

✖

Decatur Bainbridge Press
Fax: 901/454-9571
💻 DBainbrdge@aol.com

The Educated Heart
NCBTMB Home Ethics Test

Order *The Educated Heart* NCBTMB Home Ethics Test,
3 hours credit, Category A.

To order, ☎ 877/327-0600 (toll free).
Monday-Thursday, 9 a.m. to 5 p.m. (CST).
Major Credit Cards accepted.

*Nina McIntosh is approved by the National Certification Board for Therapeutic Massage
and Bodywork (NCBTMB) as a continuing education provider under Category A.*

www.educatedheart.com